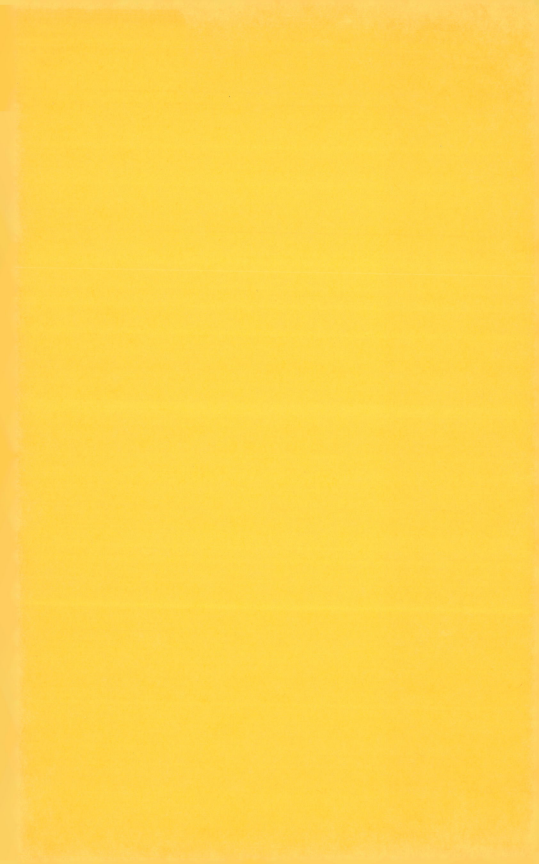

**Is Prevention Better
Than Cure?**

Studies in Social Economics

TITLES PUBLISHED

STUDIES IN SOCIAL ECONOMICS

Louise B. Russell

Is Prevention Better Than Cure?

THE BROOKINGS INSTITUTION
Washington, D.C. 20036

RA427
R87
1986

Library of Congress Cataloging-in-Publication data:
Russell, Louise B.
  Is prevention better than cure?
  (Studies in social economics)
  Includes bibliographical references and index.
    1. Medicine, Preventive—Evaluation.   2. Medicine,
Preventive—Cost effectiveness.   3. Medical economics.
4. Medicine, Preventive—United States—Evaluation.
5. Medicine, Preventive—United States—Cost effectiveness.
6. Medical economics—United States.   I. Title.   II. Series.
RA427.R87   1986   338.4'3613   85-21250
ISBN 0-8157-7632-2
ISBN 0-8157-7631-4 (pbk.)

9 8 7 6 5 4 3 2 1

THE BROOKINGS INSTITUTION is an independent organization devoted to nonpartisan research, education, and publication in economics, government, foreign policy, and the social sciences generally. Its principal purposes are to aid in the development of sound public policies and to promote public understanding of issues of national importance.

The Institution was founded on December 8, 1927, to merge the activities of the Institute for Government Research, founded in 1916, the Institute of Economics, founded in 1922, and the Robert Brookings Graduate School of Economics and Government, founded in 1924.

The Board of Trustees is responsible for the general administration of the Institution, while the immediate direction of the policies, program, and staff is vested in the President, assisted by an advisory committee of the officers and staff. The by-laws of the Institution state: "It is the function of the Trustees to make possible the conduct of scientific research, and publication, under the most favorable conditions, and to safeguard the independence of the research staff in the pursuit of their studies and in the publication of the results of such studies. It is not a part of their function to determine, control, or influence the conduct of particular investigations or the conclusions reached."

The President bears final responsibility for the decision to publish a manuscript as a Brookings book. In reaching his judgment on the competence, accuracy, and objectivity of each study, the President is advised by the director of the appropriate research program and weighs the views of a panel of expert outside readers who report to him in confidence on the quality of the work. Publication of a work signifies that it is deemed a competent treatment worthy of public consideration but does not imply endorsement of conclusions or recommendations.

The Institution maintains its position of neutrality on issues of public policy in order to safeguard the intellectual freedom of the staff. Hence interpretations or conclusions in Brookings publications should be understood to be solely those of the authors and should not be attributed to the Institution, to its trustees, officers, or other staff members, or to the organizations that support its research.

Foreword

Prevention is opening up exciting new possibilities for improving health. Over the last several decades new vaccines, screening techniques, and other preventive measures have been developed and proven effective. An impressive amount of evidence has accumulated that personal habits such as smoking, exercise, and diet play an important role in health. In response to these new possibilities, Americans are jogging, changing their menus, taking medication for high blood pressure, and making other changes in the way they live that, together, amount to a health revolution.

The beneficial effects of prevention on health are increasingly well known, but its costs and risks are not as clear. These dimensions, too, need to be assessed. Making good choices in health, as in other fields, requires consideration of the full range of outcomes—health benefits, health risks, and resource costs. In an era when containing medical costs has become a serious concern, it is particularly important to choose wisely in order to gain the most health from our limited resources. We need better evaluations of prevention to ensure that it receives a reasonable share of resources and that those resources are allocated to the most effective preventive programs.

In this book, Louise B. Russell examines the policy debates about several preventive measures—the smallpox and measles vaccines, drug therapy for high blood pressure, and exercise—to demonstrate the many complex factors involved in evaluating them. For these and other preventive measures, the evidence indicates that they rarely reduce medical expenditures. Thus prevention is not the answer to rising health care costs. Instead it offers better health at additional cost, squarely posing the question: when is the health gain worth the cost? Using the case studies, the volume explains the methods of cost-effectiveness analysis, methods that can contribute toward the balanced and complete evaluations necessary to answer the question. These methods assume a new importance in the more cost-conscious climate in which medical care now takes place. The author proposes an agenda to make them still more helpful to the decisions ahead.

Louise B. Russell is a senior fellow in the Brookings Economic Studies program. She benefited from the opportunity to present some of the conclusions of the study at a symposium on the value of preventive medical care sponsored by the Ciba Foundation in London, England, April 10–12, 1984. She is particularly grateful to Jan Blanpain, who first encouraged the foundation to consider such a symposium. The study itself was financed with the help of a grant from the National Center for Health Services Research, part of the Department of Health and Human Services. Jean Carmody monitored the project for the National Center.

The author is grateful to Kenneth Warner, whose illuminating comments on an early project paper were important in shaping the study's conclusions. The full manuscript was reviewed by Alice Rivlin, Donald Berwick, Allan Detsky, Fred Hellinger, and two anonymous reviewers. All of them provided comments that helped the author improve the substance as well as the style and clarity of the manuscript.

She also thanks Susan F. Woollen for preparing the footnotes and handling the word processing of the manuscript; the Brookings library staff for tracking down the source material; and Joy Robinson, Patricia J. Regan, and Janet Chakarian for research assistance. Jeanette Morrison edited the manuscript, Carolyn Rutsch checked it for factual accuracy, and Diana Regenthal prepared the index.

The views expressed in this study are the author's and should not be ascribed to the officers, trustees, or other staff members of the Brookings Institution, to the National Center for Health Services Research, or to any of those who were consulted or who commented on the manuscript.

BRUCE K. MAC LAURY
President

November 1985
Washington, D.C.

Contents

chapter one Introduction

Prevention of disease has brought many gains in health and life expectancy during this century. In the United States, diseases that were major causes of death in 1900, such as tuberculosis, typhoid, diphtheria, and gastroenteritis, have virtually disappeared. Much of the credit goes to public health measures, particularly purer water and food and better handling of sewage, and to higher standards of living, which brought better nutrition, housing, and personal hygiene. Thanks to these improvements, people are less often exposed to disease and better able to withstand it when they are exposed. Vaccines, a few of them quite old, have helped control some diseases: smallpox vaccine was developed in 1796 and both the vaccine and techniques for administering it had greatly improved by the early decades of the twentieth century; a vaccine for use against diphtheria was also available by 1900.[1] Advances in medical therapy, especially antibiotics, have also been important in bringing many of the infectious diseases under control.

The major causes of death now are the chronic, degenerative diseases of middle and old age. As experience with these diseases accumulates, it becomes increasingly clear that they too can often be prevented, or at least delayed for many years. Waiting until a disease is obvious and then trying to treat it is not the only option. At the same time, recent discoveries such as the vaccines against measles and rubella continue to improve our ability to prevent infectious diseases.

These possibilities have generated a new surge of interest in prevention in the United States and elsewhere. In 1979 the surgeon general of the United States published *Healthy People . . . [A] Report on Health Promotion and Disease Prevention*, which represented an "emerging consensus among scientists and the health community that the Nation's

1. Carl C. Dauer, Robert F. Korns, and Leonard M. Schuman, *Infectious Diseases* (Harvard University Press, 1968).

1

health strategy must be dramatically recast to emphasize the prevention of disease."[2] It was followed in 1980 by a report, *Promoting Health, Preventing Disease*, which set out specific objectives for improving the health of the population.[3] The same year a Canadian task force published a major report recommending "health protection packages" for each stage of life—combinations of screening tests, vaccinations,[4] and counseling to prevent disease or catch it early.[5] Educational campaigns to encourage people to exercise, quit smoking, and adopt other healthy practices have been launched in several European countries.[6]

The appeal of prevention is straightforward. Clearly, it is better not to suffer a disease than to have it and try to repair the damage afterwards. By avoiding the disease, an individual avoids the pain and suffering that accompany it, and the suffering of relatives and friends who would care for and worry about the sick person. And then, it may not be possible to repair the damage completely, or at all—the sick person may die or be left with a permanent disability of some kind.

Some people have argued that, in addition to its obvious benefits, prevention costs less than cure. The cost of many preventive measures—for example, vaccinations and many screening tests—is rather small. Smokers pay good money for cigarettes, nonsmokers do not. When disease is prevented, the costs of treating it are also avoided, so there are savings to be balanced against any costs of prevention. Many people believe that those savings are so great that more attention should be given to prevention simply on the ground that it saves money.[7]

In reality the situation is more complicated than these expectations,

2. Department of Health, Education, and Welfare, *Healthy People: The Surgeon General's Report on Health Promotion and Disease Prevention* (Government Printing Office, 1979), p. vii.

3. Department of Health and Human Services, *Promoting Health, Preventing Disease: Objectives for the Nation* (GPO, Fall 1980).

4. Today the term *vaccination* is generally applied to the use of a vaccine in order to produce immunity to a disease, although in its older usage it applied more specifically to vaccination against smallpox. The more inclusive term *immunization* refers simply to the production of immunity in individuals by any means.

5. Health and Welfare Canada, *Periodic Health Examination: Report of a Task Force to the Conference of Deputy Ministers of Health* (Ottawa, 1980).

6. Brian Abel-Smith and Alan Maynard, *The Organization, Financing and Cost of Health Care in the European Community*, Social Policy Series 36 (Brussels: Commission of the European Communities, 1979).

7. For example, in his foreword to *Healthy People*, President Jimmy Carter wrote that prevention "can substantially reduce both the suffering of our people and the burden on our expensive system of medical care."

which are reasonable on their face, would suggest. Preventing disease involves risks as well as benefits, although the risks are usually low. And even when the financial cost of the preventive measure looks small, careful evaluation often shows that the full costs are rather large, larger than any savings. In fact, prevention usually adds to medical expenditures.

The recent debate over whooping cough vaccine is a good example of the problem of risks.[8] The controversy flared in the early 1970s, after routine vaccination of children had been practiced for many years, because the evidence accumulating from several European studies showed that vaccination was occasionally associated with serious neurologic illnesses, which in some cases were followed by permanent brain damage. These reports led many parents to refuse to allow their children to be vaccinated. Their fears were increased by studies casting doubt on the vaccine's effectiveness. In Sweden public and professional confidence fell so low that whooping cough vaccine was officially withdrawn in 1979.

As a result of the controversy, new studies were undertaken to determine more carefully whether the vaccine had the effects claimed, and how often they occurred. The National Childhood Encephalopathy Study, a British program, concluded that there is a risk associated with whooping cough vaccine, but that earlier studies had overstated the size of the risk. Data from this study put the true figure in the range of one serious neurologic disorder within seven days of vaccination for every 44,000 to 360,000 children vaccinated.[9] Follow-up showed that most of the sick children recovered completely, with no signs of permanent damage. The authors of one review conclude, from these data and others, that the health benefits of the vaccine outweigh its risks. They note, however, that parents and doctors who share their conclusion must be willing to "accept the fact that active preventive measures, such as

8. D. L. Miller, R. Alderslade, and E. M. Ross, "Whooping Cough and Whooping Cough Vaccine: The Risks and Benefits Debate," *Epidemiologic Reviews*, vol. 4 (1982), pp. 1–23.

9. Enormous sample sizes are required to estimate the probability of such rare events precisely; for very rare events, nothing less than the entire population will do. The National Childhood Encephalopathy Study used a case-control design. It included all cases of children aged 2 months to 3 years hospitalized for acute neurologic illness between mid-1976 and mid-1979, and compared them with a group of control children, two matched to each case, to determine whether those with illness were more likely to have been vaccinated during the week just preceding the illness. Ibid., p. 19.

pertussis [whooping cough] immunization, sometimes carry unavoidable risks which have to be weighed against the risks of allowing nature to take its course."[10]

The detection and treatment of high blood pressure (also called hypertension) illustrate how misleading incomplete statements about cost can be.[11] Few things are cheaper than a blood pressure test. The low cost per test, and the high cost of treating the heart attacks and strokes that often result from hypertension, suggest that detecting and treating hypertension would reduce medical expenditures. But a complete accounting of costs gives a different picture. First, current recommendations are that all adults should have their blood pressure checked every year or two; thus the cost of testing the population is substantial even though the cost per test is small. Further, this expenditure produces no health benefits since, by itself, the test does nothing to improve health. Anyone whose pressure is high on the first test must be retested several times over weeks or months to be sure that the first result was not simply a fluke. If the diagnosis is confirmed, the patient must be evaluated more thoroughly before treatment is prescribed, another expense. Treatment usually involves drugs, which the patient must take regularly for many years to keep his or her blood pressure under control; the cost of drugs averages several hundred dollars a year.

Some savings result from treating hypertension because patients who take drugs faithfully will, on average, suffer less illness than those with untreated hypertension. But it turns out that the cumulative medical costs of treating hypertension are far larger than the savings. In a classic study, Weinstein and Stason estimated that, for people with moderate or severe hypertension, the costs of treating hypertension are four times as large as the savings.[12] For people with mild hypertension, the costs were more than six times the savings. Thus despite the low cost of the initial test, treating hypertension adds more to medical expenditures than it saves.[13]

10. Ibid., p. 22.

11. Hypertension detection and treatment are discussed at length in chapter 3.

12. Milton C. Weinstein and William B. Stason, *Hypertension: A Policy Perspective* (Harvard University Press, 1976), p. 60; and Weinstein and Stason, "Economic Considerations in the Management of Mild Hypertension," *Annals of the New York Academy of Sciences*, vol. 304 (March 30, 1978), pp. 424–40. They included only the costs of an initial test for everyone, not the costs of regular annual tests.

13. Employers would want to know as well whether they might expect additional savings from reduced absenteeism. Using the same approach and much of the same

As these examples show, first impressions about something as complicated as preventive care can prove incomplete in important ways, or flatly wrong. There are simply too many factors involved. It takes considerable information, thought, and care to arrive at correct conclusions about

—whether, considering risks as well as beneficial effects, a preventive measure improves health in the first place;

—how much the measure costs, with due allowance for any savings;

—and finally, whether the health benefits represent a reasonable return for the money.

At any time, it is important to evaluate major investments carefully, whether they are investments in prevention or something else. Resources are limited and there are always more good ways to use them than there are resources to use. Thus it is important to know whether a specific investment in prevention is a better use of resources than other possible investments, particularly alternative investments in health. To decide this, it is essential to know the benefits and costs of the investment and how those compare with the benefits and costs of alternative investments.

In addition, there are special reasons to consider the evaluation of prevention at this time. Renewed popular and professional interest is one reason. Proposals to make important changes in the lives and medical care of millions of people deserve careful evaluation. The claims being made for prevention as a way to cut medical costs are another reason. These claims have attracted considerable attention because of concern over the growth in national medical expenditures. If the claims are generally untrue, and the available evidence indicates they are, they may lead to an unwarranted disenchantment with prevention. For even when prevention does not save money, it can be a worthwhile investment in better health, and this—not cost saving—is the criterion on which it should be judged.

This study is about evaluating prevention. It serves two major purposes. First, it reviews the facts about some important preventive measures, and the results of careful evaluations of these measures. Second, it describes, promotes, and helps improve the principles of cost-

---

data as Weinstein and Stason, Hannan and Graham show the reductions would have to be far greater than any that have been observed to offset the added medical costs. See Edward L. Hannan and Kenneth Graham, "A Cost-Benefit Study of a Hypertension Screening and Treatment Program at the Work Setting," *Inquiry*, vol. 15 (December 1978), pp. 345–57.

effectiveness analysis on which the evaluations are based. These principles describe how to sum up the health effects of a measure and its financial costs, and compare them. While the evaluation of prevention has much in common with the evaluation of other investments, it presents some special and interesting difficulties: how to represent health benefits; how to trace through the sometimes complicated chain of events from prevention to health effect; how to deal with the particular importance of timing in the assessment of preventive care; and more. These issues are brought up in the context of the preventive measures that illustrate them best.[14]

The study focuses primarily on preventive measures that fall within the traditional boundaries of medical care. Many effective forms of prevention are excluded by these boundaries—safety at work and on the highways, further improvements in water and sewage systems, control of air pollution, and others. These can be evaluated by the same principles and in some instances have been.[15]

Chapter 2 considers two examples of the strategy of vaccination: smallpox and measles vaccines. Chapter 3 discusses the evaluation of screening tests, using screening for hypertension as the major example and bringing in cancer screening briefly at the end of the chapter. Chapter 4 steps a bit beyond medical care and looks at the evaluation of changes in lifestyle; the specific example in this chapter is exercise.

Evaluations are necessarily comparative—how does this preventive investment compare with an alternative use of resources? In most calculations, the alternative is acute medical care, or more precisely, the alternative is to do nothing until the disease appears and then to use whatever therapies are available to combat it. Less often, the alternative is another preventive strategy. For the most part, then, the evaluations discussed in this book compare preventive and acute care. Thus they directly address an issue that has become prominent in the debate over medical policy in recent years, the issue of whether the United States

---

14. Cost-effectiveness analysis has the same aim as cost-benefit analysis—to calculate and compare the costs and benefits of a proposed action. The difference is that cost-benefit analysis values all outcomes, including health effects, in dollars, while cost-effectiveness analysis measures health effects separately and in terms of units more natural to them, such as lives saved.

15. See, for example, James C. Miller III and Bruce Yandle, eds., *Benefit-Cost Analyses of Social Regulation: Case Studies from the Council on Wage and Price Stability* (Washington, D.C.: American Enterprise Institute for Public Policy Research, 1979).

and other countries are investing too much in acute care and not enough in prevention. This issue is examined further in the fifth and final chapter, after the evidence of the intervening chapters has been presented.

Pulling together the threads that run through the earlier chapters, chapter 5 discusses the conclusions that can be drawn from the evaluations of prevention in the literature. One principal conclusion is that, even among the best studies, there is considerable variation in approach and even some disagreement on basic principles. If evaluations are to be as useful as they can be, by allowing fair comparisons across a range of preventive and acute care investments, they must adopt a more standardized approach. The chapter suggests some standards and touches on remaining areas of controversy.

Each chapter begins with the discussion of specific preventive measures—or, in the last chapter, of conclusions about a range of measures—and presents the facts, the issues, and the history of the policy debates. Toward the end of each chapter the methods and results of cost-effectiveness analysis are presented. Some readers may find these later sections a bit technical. Those who do or who are primarily interested in the policy debates can skim these sections, focusing on the results of the studies and skipping the details of the methods.

A simple checklist of items—populations and frequency, size of risks, uncertainty of risks, individual values, and time—helps bring out why the full story about a preventive measure is often different from first impressions.

Populations and frequency. The costs of a preventive program depend on the size of the population at risk, while its health benefits derive from the smaller number who, in its absence, would actually have contracted the disease. By contrast, only those with the disease incur the costs of acute care and they also derive its health benefits. As a result, the costs per person of acute care can be much higher than those of prevention and still produce the same, or even lower, costs per life saved, or per year of life saved.

The frequency with which a preventive measure must be repeated has a similar effect on costs and benefits. For example, screening tests for high blood pressure, cancer, or other diseases must be repeated at regular intervals if they are to detect disease early enough to be helpful. Each repetition must be applied to the entire population at risk, only a few of whom will be found to have the disease at a given screening.

Size of risks. The most important risk, the risk of contracting disease, is implicit in the discussion of populations. Since the risk of getting the disease is usually considerably less than 100 percent, the population that will need acute care is considerably smaller than the population that needs the preventive measure. But there are other important risks. The ones most frequently overlooked are those associated with the preventive measure itself—the possibility that a vaccine will harm the recipient, or that a screening test will lead to misdiagnosis. Acute care also has risks, but these affect a smaller number of people.

Uncertainty of risks. The available information about risks, both those of the disease and of the preventive and therapeutic means of combating it, seldom allows precise estimates of those risks. If the estimates are very imprecise, it may not even be clear which is riskier, the disease or the preventive measure. But even a clearly lower risk for prevention does not mean that prevention is preferable, since more people are subject to it than to the disease and since the people who suffer from the preventive measure may not be the same ones who would have suffered from the disease. These issues become more important the more uncertain the estimates of risk.

Individual values. The true benefit of any preventive action is not the objective improvements in length of life and in health, but the value individuals place on those improvements, and how they value them in comparison with alternative outcomes. For example, data from clinical trials of antihypertensive drugs can show that they cause drowsiness and fatigue but cannot show whether those side effects are worth the probable gain in length of life. Similarly, objective data cannot show whether the likely side effects from an influenza vaccination are worth the reduction in the probability of getting flu. These judgments depend on individual preferences—and on individual responses to prevention, since not everyone experiences the same effects—and may vary from one individual to another, leading some to decide in favor of the measure, others against.

Time. Prevention must be undertaken before, sometimes long before, the disease would appear. The length of time between adoption of a preventive measure and the payoff in health is clearly important. Even small costs suffered now, and these include physical and psychological costs as well as financial ones, can weigh heavily against the possibility that disease will be prevented in the distant future. By contrast, the person in need of acute care feels unwell and may be suffering from a condition expected to prove dangerous in the short term. The costs of treatment begin at once, but the benefits also follow almost immediately.

These items underlie the discussions of the information about and debates over smallpox and measles vaccines, drug treatment for hypertension, and exercise. They are used explicitly at the conclusion of each chapter to emphasize some of the points in the chapter and to suggest briefly how other preventive measures differ from the longer cases.

chapter two **Vaccination**

Vaccination is one of the oldest and best known of the scientific methods of prevention. By inducing the production of antibodies, a vaccine creates an immunity that protects the individual against disease.

The two vaccines discussed in this chapter illustrate the general point that no preventive intervention is static. As the intervention changes, and as the conditions in which it is applied change, its value must be reassessed. Smallpox vaccine offers a unique example of this fact because its long history, culminating in the eradication of the disease in the 1970s, allowed time for the balance of risks and benefits to alter repeatedly. Each change renewed debate over the proper policy for its use. The much shorter history of measles vaccine, first available in 1963, shows the early stages of a modern vaccine's application and the evolution of policy as experience reveals new information about risks and benefits.

Smallpox

The English physician Edward Jenner developed the first vaccine, the smallpox vaccine, in 1796.[1] It arose from Jenner's observation that exposure to cowpox, a disease of cattle similar to smallpox but much milder, protected humans against smallpox. Vaccination quickly replaced the older practice of variolation, in which healthy people were

---

1. See A. B. Christie, *Infectious Diseases: Epidemiology and Clinical Practice*, 3d ed. (New York: Churchill Livingstone, 1980), chap. 9; Ralph Chester Williams, *The United States Public Health Service, 1798–1950* (Washington, D.C.: Commissioned Officers Association of the United States Public Health Service, 1951), chap. 2; and Donald R. Hopkins, *Princes and Peasants: Smallpox in History* (University of Chicago Press, 1983), chap. 1.

infected with material from smallpox sores. While variolation usually produced immunity, it sometimes produced disease instead and the variolated individual, who was highly infectious for a time, could also spread the disease to others.[2]

Smallpox vaccination arrived in the United States in 1800, when a colleague in England sent some of the new vaccine to Benjamin Waterhouse, a doctor in Boston.[3] Waterhouse tried it out on his own household and proved to his satisfaction that it worked. He then began an exchange of letters with Thomas Jefferson, which ended in his persuading Jefferson to try the vaccine in Virginia. Through Jefferson's efforts, Congress subsequently agreed that vaccination should be encouraged and in 1813 passed an act authorizing the president "to appoint an agent to preserve the genuine vaccine matter, and to furnish same to any citizen of the United States whenever it may be applied for, through the medium of the post office."[4]

Smallpox subsided for a while after the introduction of vaccination.[5] But, lulled into complacency by years of relative safety, people neglected vaccination, and the incidence of the disease rose until it was once again a serious problem. The growth of the public schools in the second half of the nineteenth century put children at particular risk and stimulated a new concern with preventing the spread of the disease. In 1855 Massachusetts became the first state to pass a law requiring that children be vaccinated against smallpox before entering school, and in 1860 New York gave local authorities the right to enforce the vaccination of school children if they chose. Many other states followed suit.[6] To prevent the introduction of new cases of smallpox from outside the country, quarantine measures were enforced against ships engaged in trade with foreign countries. Ships were quarantined if they came from ports known

2. I. Arita, "Farewell to Smallpox Vaccination," in W. Hennessen and C. Huygelen, eds., *Developments in Biological Standardization*, vol. 43: *International Symposium on Immunization: Benefit versus Risk Factors* (S. Karger, 1979), pp. 283–84.

3. Williams, *United States Public Health Service, 1798–1950*, p. 69.

4. Ibid., p. 70. The act was repealed in 1822 after a mistaken shipment of smallpox virus instead of cowpox virus caused an outbreak of disease in North Carolina. Hopkins, *Princes and Peasants*, p. 267.

5. John Duffy, "School Vaccination: The Precursor to School Medical Inspection," *Journal of the History of Medicine and Allied Sciences*, vol. 33 (July 1978), pp. 344–55.

6. Carl C. Dauer, Robert F. Korns, and Leonard M. Schuman, *Infectious Diseases* (Harvard University Press, 1968), pp. 1–9, 78–79; and Duffy, "School Vaccination."

to be infected or if crew or passengers showed signs of disease; cargo might be fumigated.[7]

The campaigns to vaccinate school children provoked considerable controversy, controversy which was continually renewed as the risks and benefits of the procedure changed.[8] Vaccination has always involved risks of its own, occasionally causing death, and not everyone was persuaded that it was effective against smallpox.[9] Organized groups and local citizens fought the passage of state laws or local regulations requiring the vaccination of school children and tried to have them repealed where they were already on the books, or at least amended to permit exceptions. And since enforcement depended on local school boards or boards of health, existing laws were often enforced loosely or not at all when there was strong community opposition.

The fortunes of vaccination waxed and waned with the disease itself. When the incidence of smallpox declined, the campaigns lagged and their opponents made headway. When fresh epidemics broke out, putting a clear threat before the community, local authorities generally succeeded in vaccinating most children, even if they were backed by nothing stronger than their own powers of persuasion. Gradually, the practice of vaccination was accepted as effective.

Around the turn of the century, the balance of risks and benefits shifted again. Smallpox was still widespread in the United States, but it began to take a milder form.[10] Throughout the 1900s, smallpox had been a severe disease with a high mortality rate; it left survivors scarred and sometimes blind. Toward the end of the century, a milder strain appeared, with much lower mortality. In the decades that followed, the severe type declined, while cases of the milder type became quite numerous.

The argument over compulsory vaccination continued as the consequences of the disease changed. Some state laws were repealed or amended.[11] Although proponents of vaccination were increasingly able to document its effectiveness,[12] they had few statistics to demonstrate

7. Williams, *United States Public Health Service, 1798–1950*, pp. 80–100.

8. Duffy, "School Vaccination," pp. 348–55.

9. See, for example, W. Asbury, "The Case against Vaccination," *Journal of the Royal Sanitary Institute*, vol. 48 (October 1927), pp. 140–56.

10. Dauer and others, *Infectious Diseases*, pp. 78–79; and Hopkins, *Princes and Peasants*, pp. 5–6. The milder form was called Variola minor, the more severe form Variola major.

11. C. C. Pierce, "Some Reasons for Compulsory Vaccination," *Boston Medical and Surgical Journal*, vol. 192 (April 9, 1925), pp. 689–95.

12. W. F. Draper, "The Occurrence of Smallpox in the United States and Measures

its safety and were inclined simply to assert that the risks were trifling and the vaccine harmless.[13] The procedure was given another push forward, however, by a number of virulent outbreaks of smallpox in the 1920s. One expert reported that "the mortality from some of the recent smallpox epidemics has reached figures which had been considered things of the past."[14] With the disease a continued threat, vaccination became still more widely applied and accepted.

At the same time vaccination was becoming a safer procedure.[15] After 1902, when the federal Public Health Service assumed responsibility for supervising the manufacture of products like smallpox vaccine, adverse reactions due to contaminated vaccine declined.[16] Through its research, the service discovered that bandages applied to the vaccination site could cause tetanus even if they were sterile, and in 1921 it recommended that none be applied. Unnecessarily large incisions also caused adverse reactions. The Public Health Service warned against this practice in 1921 and introduced a new method that produced fewer reactions, smaller scars, and a higher percentage of successful vaccinations.

By the 1930s, the incidence of smallpox was clearly falling, and falling sharply. In 1920, 110,000 cases had been reported.[17] By 1935–39, despite a brief upsurge during these years, the number of reported cases averaged only 10,000 annually. In the late 1940s the average was down to about 200 a year. At this point health authorities began to check every case against strict diagnostic criteria for smallpox. The last case to meet these criteria occurred in the early 1950s.[18]

Systematic vaccination campaigns had eliminated smallpox not only in the United States but in Canada, Australia, New Zealand, Japan, and

---

Taken by the Federal Government for Its Control," *Boston Medical and Surgical Journal,* vol. 193 (September 3, 1925), pp. 466–70; Pierce, "Some Reasons for Compulsory Vaccination"; Benjamin White, "Smallpox and Vaccination," *Boston Medical and Surgical Journal,* vol. 188 (April 12, 1923), pp. 523–30; and Samuel B. Woodward, "Smallpox in the United States, Insular Possessions, New England and Massachusetts, 1913–1923," *Boston Medical and Surgical Journal,* vol. 192 (January 8, 1925), pp. 60–64.

13. J. P. Leake and John N. Force, "Smallpox and Vaccination," *Journal of the American Medical Association,* vol. 81 (September 29, 1923), pp. 1072–76; and White, "Smallpox and Vaccination."

14. Pierce, "Some Reasons for Compulsory Vaccination," p. 691. See also Draper, "Occurrence of Smallpox in the United States."

15. Williams, *United States Public Health Service, 1798–1950,* pp. 183–85.

16. Draper, "Occurrence of Smallpox in the United States," p. 470.

17. David T. Karzon, "Smallpox Vaccination in the United States: The End of an Era," *Journal of Pediatrics,* vol. 81 (September 1972), p. 601.

18. Dauer and others, *Infectious Diseases,* pp. 78–79.

Europe by the early 1950s.[19] Nonetheless, because smallpox was still endemic in other parts of the world, these countries continued their quarantine systems for foreign travelers and, as a second line of defense against imported cases, their policies of routine vaccination. The recommended practice in the United States was to vaccinate all infants, to revaccinate children before they entered school, and thereafter to revaccinate people at particularly high risk, such as hospital workers or soldiers. Those exposed to smallpox during outbreaks were to be revaccinated as necessary, but definitely if the last successful vaccination was more than three years old.[20] The recommendations reflected the experience that vaccine produced a high level of immunity for at least three years, which declined thereafter until, after twenty years, very little was left, although that little was believed to reduce the chances of death if the disease was contracted. Then, as today, there was no therapy that could cure smallpox once the symptoms appeared.[21]

The situation after 1950 was thus dramatically different from what it had been in the nineteenth century, or even in the early decades of the twentieth century. Although not followed to the letter, the policy of routine vaccination and revaccination was more rigorously observed than ever before. Millions of people were vaccinated every year. Yet the risk of the disease was much less than ever before. Smallpox had been eliminated from the United States, from its largest neighbor, Canada, and from its major trading partners. The remaining risk—unknown but small—was that the disease would be brought into the country from somewhere else, a risk that loomed larger with the increased frequency and speed of international travel.

The Policy Debate, 1950s and 1960s

As the years passed with no further cases of smallpox, it became clear that the risk of imported disease was very small indeed. Some public

---

19. Arita, "Farewell to Smallpox Vaccination," p. 284.

20. American Public Health Association, *Control of Communicable Diseases in Man: An Official Report*, 8th ed. (New York: APHA, 1955), pp. 164–67.

21. Public Health Service Advisory Committee on Immunization Practices, "New Recommendations on Smallpox Vaccination," *Clinical Pediatrics*, vol. 6 (September 1967), pp. 549–51; Karzon, "Smallpox Vaccination in the United States," pp. 602–03; J. Michael Lane, J. Donald Millar, and John M. Neff, "Smallpox and Smallpox Vaccination Policy," *Annual Review of Medicine*, vol. 22 (1971), pp. 255, 266–67; and Christie, *Infectious Diseases: Epidemiology and Clinical Practice*, pp. 245, 246–47.

health experts began to point out that the risk of disease and death from the vaccine itself, while small, was very real and probably greater than the risk of disease.[22] They argued that the quarantine program, not routine vaccination, was keeping the United States free of smallpox. Despite the millions of vaccinations every year, a small proportion of the population had no immunity to the disease, and perhaps half had enough immunity to prevent its worst consequences but not enough to prevent their contracting and helping to spread it.[23] These experts argued that routine vaccination caused unnecessary harm and that selective vaccination of high-risk groups and travelers, together with the quarantine system, were sufficient protection against imported disease.

The criticism stimulated the first national studies to investigate and quantify the risks of vaccination.[24] The first survey, not published until 1967, produced data of unprecedented quality and detail about the risks of smallpox vaccination.[25] It had two parts: a survey of households conducted by the Census Bureau to estimate the total number of vaccinations given during 1963; and a search to find and confirm every case of a serious complication. Several sources were used in the search for complications—the most important was the list of recipients of vaccinia immune globulin (VIG), a therapeutic agent for treating vaccine complications. This list was maintained by the Red Cross as part of its program for providing VIG free of charge.

The complications divided into two major types: those involving the central nervous system and those involving the skin.[26] The most common complication of the central nervous system was postvaccinal encephalitis (inflammation of the brain), which sometimes ended in death, and which

22. Lane and others, "Smallpox and Smallpox Vaccination Policy"; and C. Henry Kempe, "The End of Routine Smallpox Vaccination in the United States," *Pediatrics,* vol. 49 (April 1972), pp. 489–92.

23. Lane and others, "Smallpox and Smallpox Vaccination Policy," p. 256; and Karzon, "Smallpox Vaccination in the United States," pp. 605–06.

24. Until the 1960s the only published study based on data from the United States reported the complications after a mass vaccination program in New York in 1947. That study had not distinguished between those who were being vaccinated for the first time and those who had been vaccinated at least once previously, an important omission since complications were believed to be much more frequent after primary vaccinations. John M. Neff and others, "Complications of Smallpox Vaccination: I. National Survey in the United States, 1963," *New England Journal of Medicine,* vol. 276 (January 19, 1967), p. 125.

25. Ibid., pp. 125–32.

26. In addition, there was a miscellaneous group of complications. Lane and others, "Smallpox and Smallpox Vaccination Policy," pp. 257–61.

was difficult to avoid because no way had been found to identify individuals at high risk. Skin complications comprised a variety of rashes and sometimes accompanied conditions severe enough to cause death. Serious skin complications generally occurred in individuals with eczema, other skin disorders, or a history of eczema, or in individuals with immunologic deficiencies caused by disease or therapy. Most of these complications could be avoided by not vaccinating these people, or people living in the same households, who might infect them.

The study estimated that more than 14 million vaccinations were given in the United States during 1963, a number that agreed with manufacturers' estimates of the doses distributed that year. Just over 6 million were primary vaccinations and just under 8 million were revaccinations. Seven deaths were attributed to vaccination. Including the deaths, 433 cases of serious complications were identified: 289 had received primary vaccinations; 17, revaccinations; and 86, no vaccination themselves but had been infected by a vaccinee; the vaccination status of the remaining 41 cases could not be determined. One hundred and ninety-three of the cases required hospitalization.

The results agreed with European studies in showing that serious complications occurred much more often after primary vaccinations than revaccinations — over twenty times more often. They also indicated that babies under 1 year of age suffered a rate of serious complications three times that of any other age-group. The authors concluded that the majority of the complications could have been avoided if doctors and nurses had screened more carefully for those known to be at high risk, such as those with eczema, and if they had practiced the best vaccination technique.

The first change produced by the debate was the recommendation, made by the Immunization Practices Advisory Committee of the Public Health Service in 1966, that vaccination should be delayed until the second year of life in light of the high rate of complications in the first year.[27] But at the time the committee decided in favor of continuing the policy of routine vaccination.

A second survey of serious complications was undertaken for the year 1968 and showed much the same results as the first.[28] More than 14

27. Public Health Service Advisory Committee, "New Recommendations on Smallpox Vaccination."
28. J. Michael Lane and others, "Complications of Smallpox Vaccination, 1968: National Surveillance in the United States," *New England Journal of Medicine,* vol. 281 (November 27, 1969), pp. 1201–07.

million vaccinations were given during the year—about 5.5 million primary vaccinations and 8.5 million revaccinations. A search for complications even more thorough than the earlier one turned up 572 cases, 9 of them ending in death. Again, rates of serious complications were highest among primary vaccinees and infants under 1 year of age.[29] And again, a substantial number of complications occurred among people who were not themselves vaccinated but who came into contact with those who were. The authors concluded as before that many complications could have been prevented by more careful attention to screening for high-risk individuals and to vaccination technique.

The size of the risk from vaccination was thus known with considerable certainty by the late 1960s—seven or eight deaths each year, and hundreds of serious complications, about 200 of them requiring hospitalization.[30] Thousands of mild reactions occurred as well. The difficulty was to assess the risk of a more selective vaccination policy, which could increase the chance of imported disease. No cases had been imported into the United States for twenty years, but the future might be less kind.

The proposed alternative to routine vaccination was continued quarantine combined with vaccination of health workers, military recruits, and travelers to countries where smallpox was still endemic. In the event of an importation, health workers might find themselves caring for smallpox cases before a definite diagnosis could be made and protective steps taken, and military personnel could be ordered to an endemic country without enough warning to allow vaccination before leaving. Lane, Millar, and Neff calculated that over a thirty-year period this policy would result in 60 deaths, compared with 210 under a continued policy of routine vaccination.[31] Unless importations caused at least 150 deaths, the selective policy would be better than routine vaccination. Based on the numbers of deaths during imported outbreaks in Europe, they judged that almost one importation a year would be required to cause so many deaths—a higher rate than had been true in Europe and, of course, much higher than had been true in the United States.

Considerably more uncertainty surrounded the estimates for the alternative policy than for the existing one. A troubling possibility was

29. Despite the 1966 recommendations, almost as many infants had been vaccinated as in the previous survey. Karzon, "Smallpox Vaccination in the United States," p. 602.

30. See also J. Michael Lane and others, "Deaths Attributable to Smallpox Vaccination, 1959 to 1966, and 1968," *Journal of the American Medical Association*, vol. 212 (April 20, 1970), pp. 441–44.

31. Lane and others, "Smallpox and Smallpox Vaccination Policy," pp. 266–68.

that deaths under a selective vaccination policy might be higher than estimated. Over the years, such a policy would mean that most of the adults in the high-risk groups were being vaccinated for the first time, and data from Europe indicated that serious complications might be more frequent among adult primary vaccinees than among children.[32] In particular, military recruits in the Netherlands, where childhood vaccination was no longer routine, showed a much higher rate of death and complications than had been observed among children in the United States.[33] No one could be sure that this experience was applicable to the United States, where vaccines and vaccination techniques might be somewhat different. One observer noted that the U.S. military had, over the course of twenty years, vaccinated 1 million previously unvaccinated recruits without a single death.[34] But Lane and his coauthors allowed that if the risks from vaccinating adults, or the number likely to need vaccination, were higher than their estimates, deaths from a policy of selective vaccination could equal or exceed those from the routine vaccination of children.

Complicated as it was, the argument was simplified because the participants focused on deaths in their calculations and ignored serious complications short of death. If serious complications always occurred in strict proportion to deaths—regardless of whether the vaccinees were children or adults, or whether the deaths resulted from vaccination or the disease itself—then more extensive calculations would have produced the same conclusion. In the case of smallpox, since the outcomes of vaccination and of the disease are so similar, it was perhaps unnecessary to devise some way of incorporating nonfatal complications. Where this is not the case, as in drug treatment for hypertension, it becomes imperative to weigh very different outcomes against each other (see chapter 3).

Although the costs of routine vaccination did not figure in the debate, estimates are available. The medical costs were estimated at $93 million for 1968, almost all of it for the physicians' services involved in admin-

32. Ibid., p. 267; and Public Health Service Advisory Committee, "New Recommendations on Smallpox Vaccination," p. 550.

33. Samuel L. Katz, "The Case for Continuing 'Routine' Childhood Smallpox Vaccination in the United States," *American Journal of Epidemiology*, vol. 93 (April 1971), pp. 241–44.

34. John M. Neff, "The Case for Abolishing 'Routine' Childhood Smallpox Vaccination in the United States," *American Journal of Epidemiology*, vol. 93 (April 1971), pp. 245–47.

istering the more than 14 million vaccinations given that year.[35] Adults often took time from work to be vaccinated, and future earnings were lost whenever vaccination caused disability or death; the study valued these at an additional $42 million. Both categories of expense would have been less under a policy of selective vaccination, probably substantially less. The costs of quarantine would have continued at the same level—more than $6 million estimated for traffic clearance and surveillance operations and $8 million for the time lost by the maritime industry while awaiting clearance.

The consideration that finally tipped the balance in the debate was the new, intensive effort to eradicate smallpox throughout the world begun in 1967 under the auspices of the World Health Organization. The incidence of smallpox had been declining in most countries before 1967, partly as a consequence of earlier national and international eradication efforts. As the first signs emerged that the new effort was sharply accelerating that decline, it began to appear that the risks that had been estimated for a selective policy could be taken as upper bounds.[36] They could only get lower as eradication proceeded. In 1971 the United States officially ended its policy of routine vaccination of children and adopted the more selective policy.[37]

The Eradication Effort

Several characteristics of smallpox were important in making it susceptible to eradication.[38] The victims became infectious only shortly before the distinctive rash appeared, so cases could be recognized quickly. No animal carried the disease; an intensive research effort

35. D. J. Sencer and N. W. Axnick, "Cost Benefit Analysis," in *International Symposium on Vaccination against Communicable Diseases: Proceedings of the 45th Symposium,* vol. 14, Symposia Series in Immunobiological Standardization (Basel: S. Karger, 1973), p. 39. Of this amount, $45,000 was for the institutional care of those whose reactions to the vaccine left them mentally retarded.

36. W. Charles Cockburn, "Progress in International Smallpox Eradication," *American Journal of Public Health,* vol. 56 (October 1966), pp. 1628–33; and "Smallpox Eradication: The First Significant Results," *WHO Chronicle,* vol. 23 (October 1969), pp. 465–76.

37. Kempe, "End of Routine Smallpox Vaccination," p. 489.

38. Frank Fenner, "Smallpox and Its Eradication," in N. F. Stanley and R. A. Joske, eds., *Changing Disease Patterns and Human Behaviour* (Academic Press, 1980), pp. 215–29; and Lane and others, "Smallpox and Smallpox Vaccination Policy," pp. 264–65.

during the eradication campaign turned up one pox virus in animals that could infect humans, the monkeypox, but this proved not to be a problem because it did not pass easily from one human to another. And, of course, the existence of an effective, stable vaccine was essential. The vaccine could even provide some protection to people who had already contracted the disease if it was administered early in the incubation period.

Mass vaccination campaigns led the eradication strategy.[39] Their success depended on two technological advances in particular: a freeze-dried vaccine, developed in the 1950s, which was much more stable in tropical climates than earlier forms of the vaccine; and new instruments for administering the vaccine, jet injectors and bifurcated needles, which greatly simplified the vaccination process.[40] The quality of the vaccine was, however, a serious problem in the early years of the campaign. In 1967, only 31 percent of tested batches of freeze-dried vaccine met WHO standards. WHO distributed advice on production techniques and continued to monitor vaccine quality at its two central collaborating laboratories, one in the Soviet Union and one in the United States. After 1971, more than 80 percent of the batches tested met the standard.[41]

As the campaigns progressed, the organizers learned that the containment strategy planned for later use, after mass vaccinations had reduced the incidence of disease to low levels, could be brought to bear sooner than anticipated.[42] Containment consisted of isolating cases of smallpox and vaccinating everyone within a radius of several miles of the case. It turned out that the incidence of smallpox in countries where it was still endemic was not as high as feared, making it easier to recognize new outbreaks. Further, new cases were generally infected only after close, even prolonged, contact with a sick patient. As a result, the disease spread out from its first appearance slowly and in a recognizable pattern, rather than flashing through the population. Since cases could be

39. "Smallpox Eradication: The First Significant Results."
40. Arita, "Farewell to Smallpox Vaccination," p. 284; Fenner, "Smallpox and Its Eradication," pp. 218–20; and "Smallpox Eradication: The First Significant Results," p. 475.
41. Global Commission for the Certification of Smallpox Eradication, *The Global Eradication of Smallpox: Final Report of the Global Commission for the Certification of Smallpox Eradication, December 1979* (Geneva: World Health Organization, 1980), p. 29.
42. "Smallpox Eradication: The First Significant Results," p. 474; and Fenner, "Smallpox and Its Eradication," pp. 222–23.

diagnosed almost as soon as they became infectious, it was feasible to identify an outbreak quickly and contain it. Containment became the mainstay of the campaign.

As the campaign approached its goal, emphasis shifted to searching out the last remaining cases of smallpox. Procedures for certifying the end of smallpox in each country differed with how long the country, and its neighbors, were believed to have been free of smallpox, and with the adequacy of its public health system.[43] When there was considerable uncertainty, an international commission was constituted to visit the country, not in order to track down the last cases of smallpox but to determine whether the country's own system of surveillance and reporting was capable of doing so.[44] Vaccination records and surveys were examined. Specimens were taken from patients with suspected chicken pox, which was sometimes confused with mild smallpox, and sent for laboratory confirmation. Pockmark surveys were especially important. Sample surveys of the population showing how many at each age had smallpox scars allowed the commission members to check that the country's historical records of smallpox incidence matched the physical evidence left on its population and that no cases had occurred since the last one reported.

On the basis of the evidence from countries where smallpox had been thought to be eradicated and had broken out again, WHO decided that two years without a reported case should pass before the world could be considered free of the disease.[45] In 1979 the Global Commission for the Certification of Smallpox Eradication reported that no cases had been discovered for two years. In May 1980, the World Health Assembly accepted the commission's findings and declared eradication complete.[46]

The eradication effort required an extraordinary range of modern technology.[47] The freeze-dried vaccine and new methods for administering vaccine were obviously important. Modern laboratories were essential not only for testing vaccine quality, but for testing patient specimens to confirm a diagnosis of smallpox. Inexpensive printing and photography helped publicize the campaign and inform people about

43. L. B. Brilliant and L. N. Hodakevič, "Certification of Smallpox Eradication," *Bulletin of the World Health Organization,* vol. 56, no. 5 (1978), pp. 723–33.
44. Fenner, "Smallpox and Its Eradication," pp. 225–27.
45. Ibid.
46. Global Commission, *Global Eradication of Smallpox,* pp. 11, 59.
47. See especially Fenner, "Smallpox and Its Eradication," pp. 219–20, 224–25; and "Smallpox Eradication: The First Significant Results," pp. 474–76.

procedures. Modern transportation carried health workers and members of certification commissions, as well as supplies, and modern communications allowed them to confer with each other.

It had been apparent from the outset that everyone would gain from eradication and this helped generate the exceptional international organization and cooperation required for success.[48] Each country could turn the resources previously devoted to smallpox vaccination and quarantine to other uses. Smallpox vaccination is no longer required for the general population in any country, although the U.S. armed services still vaccinate all new recruits.[49] Thus countries that had been free of indigenous smallpox for years no longer had to subject their populations to the certain risks of vaccination in order to protect them against the uncertain risks of possible importations.

With smallpox, prevention has gone through a complete and unprecedented cycle. For years before smallpox was eliminated from the United States, vaccination unquestionably made a major contribution to good health. Once the disease was eliminated, that contribution became equivocal at best. With the elimination of smallpox from the rest of the world as well, the vaccine could take credit for an unqualified success. By eliminating smallpox, it put itself out of business.

Measles

A second case will highlight more of the complications of evaluating even such a straightforward preventive measure as vaccination. Measles offers an opportunity to study the early stages of a vaccine's use more closely than smallpox because measles vaccine was first licensed in 1963, and reasonably good statistics on the disease are available for the period just before as well as after the introduction of the vaccine.

Like smallpox, measles in its natural state is a disease of childhood and virtually everyone is vulnerable.[50] It is perhaps the most highly

48. Fenner, "Smallpox and Its Eradication."
49. Confirmed by telephone with the Centers for Disease Control and the Department of State.
50. G. S. Wilson, "Measles as a Universal Disease," *American Journal of Diseases of Children,* vol. 103: *International Conference on Measles Immunization* (Bethesda, Md.: National Institutes of Health, 1962), pp. 49–53; William H. Foege, "The Global Elimination of Measles," *Public Health Reports,* vol. 97 (September–October 1982),

infectious of the infectious diseases, spreading with great speed through susceptible populations. One infection is believed to produce lifelong immunity in most people.

Statistics show that the death rate from measles dropped steadily and substantially between 1900 and 1963, although the disease continued to be virtually universal among children, with the highest attack rates among those 3 and 4 years of age.[51] In the early decades of the century deaths from measles often exceeded 100 per million total population, but by the late 1950s, the rate had dropped to 2 or 3 per million.[52]

No one really knows why deaths declined. Then as now there was no cure for the disease itself. The introduction of antibiotics, used to treat complications, and gamma globulin, which helps moderate the course of the disease, contributed to the trend.[53] Basically, however, it simply seemed to become less serious. Some hypothesize that the disease changed, others that the genetic resistance of the population to its more serious consequences increased, and still others that better nutrition and generally higher standards of living made children better able to survive the disease.[54] One investigator argues that the modern diet should receive the credit: "In the past in Europe and currently in developing countries, children could not receive sufficient energy [to survive measles] because of the bulky nature of their diet. The characteristics of bulk have been removed from the Western diet by the fine milling of cereals, removal of dietary fibres and the enormous increase in refined sugar and fats and oils."[55] His position is intriguing because he praises exactly those aspects

pp. 402–05; Christie, *Infectious Diseases: Epidemiology and Clinical Practice*, chap. 9; and Alan R. Hinman and others, "Current Features of Measles in the United States: Feasibility of Measles Elimination," *Epidemiologic Reviews*, vol. 2 (1980), pp. 153–70.

51. Wilson, "Measles as a Universal Disease"; Alexander D. Langmuir, "Medical Importance of Measles," *American Journal of Diseases of Children*, vol. 103: *International Conference on Measles Immunization* (Bethesda, Md.: National Institutes of Health, 1962), pp. 54–56; and Dauer and others, *Infectious Diseases*, p. 80.

52. See also Bureau of the Census, *Historical Statistics of the United States: Colonial Times to 1970*, vol. 1 (Government Printing Office, 1975), p. 58. On the basis of published data, deaths per 1,000 cases of measles dropped from 4 in 1935–39 to 1 in the 1950s. But these rates are overstated because many cases of measles were not reported. Dauer and others, *Infectious Diseases*, p. 80.

53. Dauer and others, *Infectious Diseases*, p. 79.

54. Christie, *Infectious Diseases: Epidemiology and Clinical Practice*, pp. 236–39, 246–47; David Morley, "Severe Measles," in Stanley and Joske, eds., *Changing Disease Patterns and Human Behaviour*, pp. 115–28; and Wilson, "Measles as a Universal Disease."

55. Morley, "Severe Measles," p. 126.

of the modern diet that have recently come in for so much criticism from other health experts.

In the years just before the vaccine was licensed, the late 1950s and early 1960s, about 500,000 cases of measles were reported every year.[56] Reporting was known to be incomplete. Studies of immunity showed that 90 percent or more of adults were immune and thus must have had measles. This fact implied that nearly everyone was infected during childhood and that the actual number of cases must be close to the number of children born each year, putting actual cases at about 4 million annually by the early 1960s.[57]

Although the disease was mild in most children by this time, it still caused death or serious impairment in some. During the three years 1959–61, an average of 400 deaths from measles were reported every year. These deaths occurred for the most part among the approximately 4,000 children each year who developed postmeasles encephalitis; of the children who survived, 1,300 suffered mental retardation or other permanent damage to the central nervous system.[58] In addition, 5,000 children each year developed other complications, such as pneumonia or otitis media, so seriously that they had to be hospitalized.

The 1963 licensing of a measles vaccine based on live virus was eagerly awaited.[59] As soon as it became available, state health departments and private physicians acted quickly to distribute it to the public. In 1966 the federal government announced an initiative to eradicate measles and provided grants for measles vaccine to state and local health departments. The effect of these combined efforts was dramatic: reported cases of measles dropped to only 22,000 in 1968.[60]

Measles was not eliminated in this first effort. Reported cases rose

56. Dauer and others, *Infectious Diseases,* p. 80; Hinman and others, "Current Features of Measles," p. 153; and "Measles Encephalitis—United States, 1962–1979," *Morbidity and Mortality Weekly Report,* vol. 30 (July 31, 1981), pp. 362–64.

57. Norman W. Axnick, Steven M. Shavell, and John J. Witte, "Benefits Due to Immunization against Measles," *Public Health Reports,* vol. 84 (August 1969), pp. 673, 675; and Hinman and others, "Current Features of Measles," p. 154.

58. Dauer and others, *Infectious Diseases,* p. 80; Axnick and others, "Benefits Due to Immunization against Measles," pp. 673, 675; and "Measles Encephalitis—United States, 1962–1979."

59. See *American Journal of Diseases of Children,* vol. 103: *International Conference on Measles Immunization* (Bethesda, Md.: National Institutes of Health, 1962).

60. Robert B. Albritton, "Cost-Benefits of Measles Eradication: Effects of a Federal Intervention," *Policy Analysis,* vol. 4 (Winter 1978), pp. 1–21; Hinman and others, "Current Features of Measles," pp. 154–56, 166; and John J. Witte and Norman W. Axnick, "The Benefits from Ten Years of Measles Immunization in the United States," *Public Health Reports,* vol. 90 (May–June 1975), pp. 206–07.

again, peaking at 75,000 in 1971 before falling to somewhat lower levels. The rise in cases followed closely on the decline in federal funds for measles vaccine as attention turned to the newly licensed vaccine for rubella, but surveys show that the proportion of children immunized against measles remained high during the early 1970s, dropping only once, between 1969 and 1970.[61] One author has suggested that the shift in federal interest led to neglect of vaccination technique during this period.[62] The upsurge in cases may also have reflected the many children left vulnerable by several less effective practices common during the trial and error of the early years: a killed-virus vaccine was distributed until 1967, gamma globulin was sometimes administered with live-virus vaccine to reduce reactions, and when supplies were short, half doses of vaccine were sometimes given.[63] All these practices were subsequently abandoned.[64]

Experience further revealed that children under 1 year were less likely than older children to develop immunity in response to the vaccine.[65] In 1976 both the American Academy of Pediatrics and the Immunization Practices Advisory Committee of the Department of Health and Human Services recommended that children not be vaccinated against measles until 15 months, except when an outbreak of the disease made earlier vaccination advisable.

In 1978 the federal government announced a second initiative to eliminate measles from the United States.[66] The effort depended first and foremost on maintaining very high levels of immunization, a require-

61. Witte and Axnick, "Benefits from Ten Years of Measles Immunization"; and Hinman and others, "Current Features of Measles."

62. James D. Cherry, "The 'New' Epidemiology of Measles and Rubella," *Hospital Practice*, vol. 15 (July 1980), p. 51.

63. J. W. Davies, S. E. Acres, and P. V. Varughese, "Experience with Measles in Canada and the United States," *Canadian Medical Association Journal*, vol. 126 (January 15, 1982), p. 125; Alan R. Hinman and Stephen R. Preblud, "Epidemic Potential of Measles and Rubella," *Journal of American College Health Association*, vol. 29 (December 1980), pp. 105–09; and Marc A. Strassburg, Sander Greenland, and Shirley L. Fannin, "Vaccine Failures in the Epidemiology and Control of Measles," *American Journal of Public Health*, vol. 69 (October 1979), pp. 1055–57.

64. Walter A. Orenstein and others, "Current Status of Measles in the United States, 1973–1977," *Journal of Infectious Diseases*, vol. 137 (June 1978), pp. 847–53.

65. Cherry, " 'New' Epidemiology of Measles and Rubella," p. 50; and Richard G. Judelsohn, Mary Lou Fleissner, and Dennis J. O'Mara, "School-based Measles Outbreaks: Correlation of Age at Immunization with Risk of Disease," *American Journal of Public Health*, vol. 70 (November 1980), pp. 1162–65.

66. See Hinman and others, "Current Features of Measles," pp. 166–69; and Hinman and Preblud, "Epidemic Potential of Measles and Rubella," p. 105.

ment crucial for the control of measles. Studies show that, because the disease is so highly infectious, about 95 percent of the population must be successfully immunized to prevent its transmission;[67] this level tests the limits of the vaccine, which even under ideal conditions produces immunity in only 90 to 95 percent of vaccinees.[68]

To achieve high levels of immunization, health authorities put primary emphasis on the passage and strict enforcement of state laws requiring children to be vaccinated against measles before they entered school. Most states had such laws when the 1978 initiative began.[69] By 1984, all states and the District of Columbia required evidence of measles immunization before school entry—usually a physician's certificate stating that live-virus vaccine had been administered after the child's first birthday or that the child had already had measles.[70] Forty-three states and the District extended the requirement to cover all grades. These laws also allowed unvaccinated children to be excluded from school during outbreaks.[71]

By the beginning of the 1983 school year, 98 percent of the children entering kindergarten or first grade had been immunized against measles.[72] Young children are so well protected that measles now occurs more often among teenagers and young adults, who may have missed being vaccinated or been vaccinated by one of the less effective methods. The Department of Health and Human Services has increasingly urged the vaccination, sometimes revaccination, of these older groups, especially on college campuses and military bases.[73]

67. Roy M. Anderson and Robert M. May, "Directly Transmitted Infectious Diseases: Control by Vaccination," *Science,* vol. 215 (February 26, 1982), p. 1059; and "Mathematics and Measles," *The Lancet* (July 31, 1982), pp. 248–49.

68. Alan R. Hinman, A. David Brandling-Bennett, and Phillip I. Nieburg, "The Opportunity and Obligation to Eliminate Measles from the United States," *Journal of the American Medical Association,* vol. 242 (September 14, 1979), pp. 1157–62; Orenstein and others, "Current Status of Measles in the United States, 1973–1977"; and Strassburg and others, "Vaccine Failures," p. 1055.

69. Hinman and others, "Current Features of Measles," pp. 164–69.

70. Alan R. Hinman and others, "Progress in Measles Elimination," *Journal of the American Medical Association,* vol. 247 (March 19, 1982), pp. 1592–95; and "Elimination of Indigenous Measles—United States," *Morbidity and Mortality Weekly Report,* vol. 31 (October 1, 1982), pp. 517–19. Updated to 1984 with data from the Centers for Disease Control.

71. Hinman and others, "Opportunity and Obligation to Eliminate Measles from the United States."

72. "Elimination of Indigenous Measles," p. 517. Updated to 1983 with data from the Centers for Disease Control.

73. Cherry, " 'New' Epidemiology of Measles and Rubella"; Hinman and others,

The new effort did not eliminate measles by October 1982, the goal set at the beginning, but it came close and may yet succeed. In 1983, only 1,497 cases of measles were reported and in 1984, 2,534, compared with more than 13,000 and 57,000 in 1980 and 1977, respectively.[74] Thus the United States has achieved a position similar to that regarding smallpox in the late 1940s—measles has almost been eliminated from the country, but it remains endemic in much of the world, indeed in a much larger area than was true for smallpox, since only Canada and Sweden among the industrialized countries have even adopted the U.S. goal of ending the spread of the disease within their own borders.[75]

As the incidence of the disease declines, the issue of the side effects of the vaccine itself will become more important. Since measles was nearly universal when there was no vaccine, virtually everyone is at risk and is a candidate for vaccination. On average, those who accept vaccination gain if the risks of the vaccine are less than those of the disease, with due allowance for the earlier age of vaccination. In fact, of course, the risks are substantially less. While no surveys of the scope undertaken in the 1960s for smallpox vaccine have been done, the available studies indicate that serious reactions—encephalitis and death—occur at the rate of 1 per million children vaccinated.[76] This compares with approximately 1,000 cases of encephalitis and 100 deaths for every million cases of measles.[77]

A British study tracked 10,035 children who received measles vaccine between 1970 and 1980 to learn more about the incidence of less serious

"Opportunity and Obligation to Eliminate Measles from the United States," pp. 1157–58; and Orenstein and others, "Current Status of Measles in the United States, 1973–1977," p. 852.

74. "Measles Going, Going...," *The Lancet* (October 16, 1982), pp. 887–88. Updated to 1984 with data from the Centers for Disease Control. Note that reporting is more complete now than it was in the 1950s and 1960s.

75. "Mathematics and Measles."

76. Cherry, " 'New' Epidemiology of Measles and Rubella," p. 49; and Orenstein and others, "Current Status of Measles in the United States, 1973–1977," p. 850. The estimate of serious reactions is based on reactions reported to the Centers for Disease Control plus additional cases reported in the literature and is likely to be an undercount.

77. The base for these rates is estimated actual cases of measles, not reported cases, which, as discussed earlier, are known to be incomplete. The rates are those observed during the late 1950s and early 1960s and may overestimate those that would have occurred without vaccination in the 1970s and later years because they make no allowance for the possibility that the long-term decline in deaths from measles would have continued.

side effects.[78] Seventy-one percent of the children were entirely well during the two weeks after vaccination. Another 28 percent had mild or moderate symptoms, usually a feeling of unwellness accompanied by fever for two or three days, less often a rash; some of the children suffered other symptoms, such as diarrhea, vomiting, or, rarely, ear infection. One percent of the children, 110 in number, experienced symptoms described as severe. One child died and twelve others were admitted to hospitals. Convulsion was the most frequent reason for admission. All the children with convulsions recovered and had no further neurological problems. The study noted that half the children with convulsions had a personal or family history of convulsions, and that such children should receive immune gamma globulin along with the vaccine. Finally, the study noted that symptoms clustered between the fifth and tenth days after vaccination, indicating that they were truly a result of the vaccination and not unrelated chance illnesses. Side effects of this magnitude are unlikely to become a major issue as long as the disease is still present. Indeed, the issue can never take the form it did with smallpox because measles is so infectious that it is highly improbable quarantine could prevent it from entering the United States.

The imminence of eradication in the United States has raised the possibility of worldwide eradication. As with smallpox, this would simultaneously eliminate both the problems caused by the disease and those caused by the vaccine. Some public health experts urge that worldwide eradication is now both feasible and desirable.[79]

The experts point out that, like smallpox, measles is fairly easy to diagnose, is not transmitted by animals, and is not carried by healthy people, characteristics that make it easy to identify and isolate.[80] Measles vaccine is now available in a freeze-dried form that remains potent for several weeks even in the heat and humidity of tropical climates. An organizational vehicle for eradication already exists in the Expanded Immunization Program of the World Health Organization, a program aimed at making several vaccines for childhood diseases, including measles vaccine, available to all the children of the world by 1990.

78. Christine L. Miller, "Surveillance after Measles Vaccination in Children," *The Practitioner,* vol. 226 (March 1982), pp. 535–37.

79. Foege, "Global Elimination of Measles"; and Donald R. Hopkins and others, "The Case for Global Measles Eradication," *The Lancet* (June 19, 1982), pp. 1396–98.

80. Davies and others, "Experience with Measles in Canada," p. 123; Foege, "Global Elimination of Measles," p. 402; and Hopkins and others, "Case for Global Measles Eradication," p. 1396.

Measles is a more serious disease in developing countries than in the industrialized nations.[81] The death rate during the first few weeks averages 5 to 7 percent, even higher in very poor areas, and it is a major cause of blindness as well as retardation among the survivors. A study of outbreaks in rural West Africa discovered that the death toll from measles continued to mount after the disease itself had passed. In the year following the outbreaks, 15 percent of the children who had had measles died, compared with 1 percent of the children who had not had the disease.[82] One medical journal notes, however, that "it has been hard to show mortality reductions from [measles] immunization in developing countries, perhaps because the children who die are so seriously undernourished or sick from other causes."[83] Thus, while eradication would improve health and save lives in developing countries, the gains might not be as large as they would appear at first glance.

Measles has, however, several characteristics that will make it more difficult to eradicate than smallpox.[84] Chief among these is its highly infectious nature, requiring the vaccination of more than 90 percent of any given population to end the spread of measles in that population. By contrast, containment turned out to be an effective weapon against the more slowly spreading smallpox and was successful even in areas where less than half the population had been vaccinated.

Achieving such high levels of vaccination will be difficult because measles occurs at much younger ages in developing countries than smallpox did, or than measles did in developed countries before the vaccine.[85] By the recommended age for vaccination in the United States—15 months—it is estimated that more than a third of the children in developing countries have already had measles.[86] Yet studies in the United States show the vaccine is less effective in infants under 1 year of age and may be essentially ineffective before the age of 6 months. The West African study concluded that vaccination was as effective at 9 months as later, supporting the WHO recommendation that infants in

81. See Foege, "Global Elimination of Measles," pp. 404–05; and Morley, "Severe Measles," pp. 119–20, 124, 126–27.

82. Harry F. Hull, Pap John Williams, and Fred Oldfield, "Measles Mortality and Vaccine Efficacy in Rural West Africa," The Lancet (April 30, 1983), pp. 972–75.

83. "Rationalising Measles Vaccination," The Lancet (August 1, 1981), pp. 236–37.

84. Foege, "Global Elimination of Measles," p. 405; and Hopkins and others, "Case for Global Measles Eradication," pp. 1396–97.

85. Foege, "Global Elimination of Measles," p. 405.

86. Morley, "Severe Measles," p. 127.

developing countries be vaccinated at 9 months, but that it was mark-
edly less effective when administered between 6 and 8 months. Thus
the eradication of measles will require intensive and frequent vaccination campaigns that reach most of the susceptible population each
time. Intensive campaigns are costly and difficult in countries with
few established health services, and as one author observes, "the cost
of reaching the last 10 or 25% of the target is disproportionately
high."[87]

Further, unlike smallpox, neither measles nor measles vaccine leaves
scars so it will be considerably more difficult to know who has been
vaccinated, or had the disease, and who remains susceptible. Either
records must be kept, an onerous burden in countries where such
recordkeeping is not routine, or serological surveys of the population
must be undertaken to determine by blood test who is immune.

The call for worldwide eradication has not yet been taken up. If the
United States, Canada, and Sweden succeed in eliminating measles
within their borders, the case will be stronger. But even then worldwide
eradication may have to await solutions for the formidable problems
posed by measles.

Summarizing Costs and Benefits

By the time analysts began to calculate the costs and benefits of
smallpox vaccination for the United States, the disease had been
eliminated, leaving only a few items to be considered. The costs consisted
of the financial outlays for routine vaccination and quarantine and the
adverse health effects of the vaccine—the deaths and disability it caused.
The benefits were difficult to calculate but simple to state: protection
from the possibility that smallpox would enter the United States from
outside. The balancing of costs and benefits could be done rather easily,
without the aid of a summary device.

Measles presents a more complicated case to evaluate and thus is
more typical than smallpox. Since the disease is still present, the number
of items in an evaluation is considerably larger. As a result, it is essential

87. W. A. M. Cutting, "Cost-Benefit Evaluations of Vaccination Programmes," *The
Lancet* (September 20, 1980), p. 634.

to have a framework for setting out the different items and combining them in ways that help show which alternative is preferable. Cost-effectiveness analysis provides such a framework.[88]

Cost-effectiveness analysis is a set of methods for answering the questions: What will this investment cost? And what effects will it have? The distinctive feature of cost-effectiveness analysis is that it shows as financial outlays only those items that are readily measured in dollars and presents health effects in units more natural to them. The results of an analysis are often summarized in terms of the financial outlay per unit of health benefit—for example, the cost per life saved. Traditional cost-benefit analysis, by contrast, attempts to value everything, including health effects, in terms of dollars. If one accepts the values used to translate health effects into dollars, this approach makes it easier to compare alternatives. But many people object to the idea that human lives and health can be represented by dollars, and even those who accept the principle, recognizing that such valuations are implicit in decisions about how to use limited resources, do not always agree on what value should be used.

Table 2-1 presents estimates from a cost-effectiveness analysis of measles vaccination published in 1969 for the years 1963–68, the first five years after the vaccine was licensed.[89] The table is a balance sheet comparing two alternatives: the extensive programs undertaken during this period to vaccinate children against measles; and no vaccination at all.[90] The effects of each alternative are divided into the categories just discussed: financial effects, or costs; and health effects. The analysis applies to the entire United States.

---

88. Kenneth E. Warner and Bryan R. Luce, *Cost-Benefit and Cost-Effectiveness Analysis in Health Care: Principles, Practice, and Potential* (Ann Arbor, Mich.: Health Administration Press, 1982); and Milton C. Weinstein and William B. Stason, "Foundations of Cost-Effectiveness Analysis for Health and Medical Practices," *New England Journal of Medicine*, vol. 296 (March 31, 1977), pp. 716–21.

89. Axnick and others, "Benefits Due to Immunization against Measles." A second analysis was done after the measles vaccine had been in use for ten years: Witte and Axnick, "Benefits from Ten Years of Measles Immunization." The earlier study, a classic of its kind, is used here because it presents estimates in more detail and thus permits a more complete discussion of the principles of cost-effectiveness analysis.

90. The alternatives can be greater in number and more complex. For example, an important issue with rubella, which causes defects in unborn babies but is otherwise a mild disease, is whether it is more cost-effective to vaccinate all preschool children or only teenaged girls.

Table 2-1. Cost-Effectiveness Evaluation of Measles Vaccination for 1963–68

	In thousands of dollars		
Costs	Without vaccination (A)	With vaccination (B)	Difference (A) − (B)
Direct medical expenses			
Administration of vaccine	. . .	108,300	− 108,300
Treatment for measles cases	174,337	96,772[a]	77,565
Treatment for vaccine side effects[b]	. . .	n.a.	n.a.
Subtotal	**174,337**	**205,072**	**− 30,735**
Net expenditures for institutional care[c]			
For persons retarded by measles	499,653	298,820[a]	200,833
For persons retarded by vaccine side effects[b]	. . .	n.a.	n.a.
Total	**673,990**	**503,892**	**170,098**

	In natural units		
Health effects	Without vaccination (A)	With vaccination (B)	Difference (A) − (B)
Deaths	2,400	1,427	973
Cases of retardation			
Caused by measles	8,000	4,756[a]	3,244
Caused by vaccine side effects[b]	. . .	n.a.	n.a.
Cases hospitalized	144,000	85,620	58,380
Days lost from school or work	83,500,000	49,651,000	33,849,000

Source: Data from Norman W. Axnick, Steven M. Shavell, and John J. Witte, "Benefits Due to Immunization against Measles," *Public Health Reports,* vol. 84 (August 1969), pp. 673–80.

n.a. Not available.

a. Cases in children who were missed by the vaccination campaign and those in whom vaccination failed to produce immunity.

b. No estimates of these costs were reported in the study. If the vaccine rarely produces serious side effects, as some current evidence suggests, the addition of these costs and health effects would not change the estimates shown in the table by very much.

c. Cost of institutional care in excess of normal maintenance costs for a person at home. Instead, the estimate should be the cost of institutional care less the *total* living expenses of a person at home. The estimate shown here is probably higher than the correct number.

Costs

Two types of financial outlay have been estimated for each alternative: direct medical expenses; and net expenditures for institutional care. The costs of not vaccinating are estimated on the assumption that measles cases would have continued to occur in the same numbers as they did in the years just before 1963.[91] They include medical treatment—about half

91. The estimate used, 4 million cases a year, is based on the number of births

of all children with measles saw a doctor and serious cases sometimes required hospitalization—and lifetime institutionalization for children left retarded by measles.

The costs of vaccinating comprise administration of the vaccine, the cost of treatment of cases of measles among children who were missed by the vaccination campaign and those in whom the vaccine failed to produce immunity, and institutionalization for any of these children left retarded by the disease. The estimates should also include the costs of treating side effects and retardation caused by the vaccine, but no estimates of these costs were made in the study.

The expenditures for long-term institutional care are estimated net of normal maintenance costs because the analysis adopts the most general perspective, and the one most often adopted for public policy, that of the society as a whole. From this perspective, the outlay estimates should not include costs that are offset by savings elsewhere, but only those that represent additional costs to society. Since a child must be fed, housed, and clothed whether it lives at home or in an institution, only the extra costs of institutionalization should be counted in the analysis. Although the estimates shown in table 2-1 are on the right track conceptually, they are probably too high, since the net cost of long-term institutionalization should be calculated as the cost over and above the average *total* expenditure for a normal child.[92]

The direct medical expenditures shown in the table are simply the sum of the expenditures in each of the years 1963 through 1968. The costs of institutionalization represent expenditures stretching many years into the future—children retarded by measles are assumed to require institutional care for an average of forty years. As is the usual practice, these future outlays have been discounted before being added, to reflect the fact that the expenditure of a dollar several years from now is not the same as the expenditure of a dollar today. For example, at a 4 percent rate of interest (over inflation), an investment of 89 cents today would yield one dollar in three years' time. Thus, at that rate of interest,

---

annually during the early 1960s. It is probably an overestimate for the period 1963–68, since births dropped below 4 million after 1964.

92. Total expenditure includes normal maintenance costs *plus* outlays for education, vacations, piano lessons, toys, and so forth. The extent of institutionalization may also be overestimated. Not all retarded children are institutionalized for their entire lives. J. W. Bush, M. M. Chen, and D. L. Patrick, "Health Status Index in Cost Effectiveness: Analysis of PKU Program," in Robert L. Berg, ed., *Health Status Indexes* (Chicago: Hospital Research and Educational Trust, 1973), pp. 172–94.

one dollar of expenditure three years from now has a present value of 89 cents. Future outlays were discounted in this fashion, using a 4 percent rate of interest, to yield the equivalent present values and these present values were summed to the total present value of institutionalization costs shown in the table.[93]

The summarizing process begins by comparing the costs of the alternatives. The third column of the table shows that vaccination required an additional $31 million in medical expenditures compared with no vaccination, but that it reduced expenditures on institutionalization by $201 million, for an overall saving of $170 million. This estimate is probably high, since several aspects of the analysis, already mentioned, contribute to overestimating the costs of not vaccinating and underestimating those of vaccinating: the number of measles cases in the absence of vaccination is probably overestimated; the net cost of institutionalization is probably overestimated, hence the savings associated with vaccination are overestimated; and the cost of treating vaccine side effects has been omitted.

Health Effects

The health effects of the two programs are listed in the lower half of table 2-1. They include the deaths, cases of retardation, numbers of hospital admissions, and days lost from school or work under each alternative. The difference column shows that vaccination represented a gain in every case: 973 lives were saved; more than 3,000 children were spared retardation; 58,000 fewer hospital admissions occurred; and 34 million school and work days were saved.[94]

Unlike the financial outlays, the health effects are not summarized. For measles, this lack does not present a serious problem. Vaccination is clearly worth undertaking, regardless of what other health programs are under consideration, since it costs less than the status quo, when expenditures for institutionalization as well as medical care are consid-

---

93. In general, the present discounted value, P_t, of a dollar amount, A_t, to be received t years from now is $P_t = A_t/(1 + r)^t$, where r is the discount rate. The sum of a series of present values over the years 1 through n is

$$S = \sum_{t=1}^{n} P_t.$$

94. The health gains from vaccination may be overstated, since the estimates of health effects without vaccination are probably too large. See note 91.

ered, and it produces gains in every category of health effect. As in the case of smallpox, the comparison of alternatives is enormously simplified because the side effects of the vaccine mimic those of the disease, so the range of health effects is the same for the two alternatives. Cases in which the health effects are different for different alternatives, or those involving net costs, pose more problems. One solution developed by analysts is the concept of a *year of healthy life* as a common unit for measuring health effects. This concept and methods for translating different effects into equivalent years of healthy life are discussed in chapter 3.

Interpreting the Results

It was noted in the first chapter that many people urge more emphasis on preventive programs because they believe prevention will reduce medical care expenditures. Table 2-1 shows that measles vaccination increased rather than reduced medical expenses during 1963–68, even though it probably saved money overall. Indeed, if the primary concern is whether measles vaccination will raise or lower medical expenditures, the estimate in the table gives an incomplete answer. It should also include the future medical expenses of people whose lives are saved by the vaccine, since these expenses would not have been incurred had they died. Adding these expenses increases the medical outlays associated with any program that saves lives.[95]

The point deserves emphasis because of the interest in prevention as a way to constrain medical expenditures.[96] If this issue is the principal concern, the question that must be answered by the analysis is: what will the program mean for medical expenditures now and in the future? To answer this question, medical expenses in added years of life must be included along with the costs of the preventive program. But if the purpose of the analysis is instead to determine whether the program is a good investment, only the costs of the preventive program should be

95. The Office of Technology Assessment has published a cost-effectiveness study of vaccination against influenza that presents estimates of the cost per year of healthy life gained from using this vaccine with and without medical expenses in added years of life. The difference is substantial—$63 per year of healthy life when medical costs in added years of life are left out, $1,956 when they are included. Office of Technology Assessment, *Cost Effectiveness of Influenza Vaccination* (GPO, 1981), p. 4.

96. This paragraph owes much to discussions with Kenneth Warner of the University of Michigan.

counted. Added years of life involve added expenditures for food, clothes, and housing as well as medical care. None of these is relevant to deciding whether the program is a good investment. Like future earnings, which are discussed below, future medical expenses are one of the indirect consequences of the health gains from a program. While estimates of them might be presented as an elaboration of those consequences, they are not an addition to health effects.

Some people argue that additional expenditures for a preventive measure ought not to be a cause for concern if the people whose lives and health are preserved will earn enough to cover those expenses. But like future medical expenses, future earnings are only one of the consequences of the health effects of a program. Good health and longer life are valuable partly because they allow people to remain productive workers longer. There are, however, other reasons as well—the simple pleasure of being alive and healthy, the pleasure it gives to others when someone they care for is alive and well, and the value of the many unpaid activities that people ordinarily engage in. All of these are implicit in the estimates of health effects. Estimates of earnings help to describe the consequences of better health in greater detail, but they are not an addition to the health effects. To include them as a separate item is to count some of the effects twice—once as a gain in health and again as a saving to be subtracted from program costs.

Further, subtracting earnings from program costs indirectly promotes programs that help workers over those that help children or retirees. Traditional cost-benefit studies that use earnings to translate health effects into dollars have this bias, and many people strongly object to it. They should be equally on guard against the use of earnings in cost-effectiveness analysis. The implications are less obvious at first glance, but much the same.

The evaluation of measles underscores another important point: an evaluation of any program, whether for prevention or something else, should be based on *all* its direct costs and benefits. When all costs and effects are considered, measles vaccination was clearly worthwhile during 1963–68. It probably produced a saving overall despite the additional medical costs and it preserved the lives and health of many children. Even if it had not yielded savings, it might well have been judged worthwhile if the outlays were reasonable in relation to the gains in health.[97]

97. The point made in chapter 1 bears repeating here: to insist that prevention save

If a new evaluation of measles vaccine based on recent experience were done, the results would differ from those in table 2-1. Vaccination is much more complete now, and the incidence of cases has dropped so low that the health gains are much greater than they were in 1963–68 (although allowance would have to be made for the possibility that measles deaths would have continued to decline in the absence of the vaccine). The cost of administering the vaccine has been reduced as well by combining it with rubella and mumps vaccines.[98] An evaluation depends on conditions at the time it is done and if conditions change, a new evaluation will produce different results. The history of smallpox illustrates how dramatically conditions, and thus the balance of costs and benefits, can change.

Some Further Issues

Evaluations of the vaccines for smallpox and measles demonstrate many of the elements common to the evaluation of any vaccine, or of any preventive measure. But they also demonstrate that no two vaccines are exactly alike. Even for the same vaccine, the balance of benefits and costs can alter dramatically from one set of circumstances to another— as the nature of the vaccine, the disease, the vulnerable population, or the medical services already available change. Vaccines other than those for smallpox and measles pose an even wider range of interesting issues. A brief review of some of these issues will help to make the point that each preventive measure must be evaluated separately and, often, reevaluated as conditions change. The review is organized around the factors listed in the first chapter and discussed in the cases of smallpox and measles—populations and frequency, risk, uncertainty, individual values, and time.

With smallpox and measles, the entire *population* is (or was) at substantial risk for serious harm from the disease. Further, the required *frequency* of vaccination against smallpox and measles is low. Vaccine is administered at most only a few times during a lifetime, making widespread prevention relatively easy and inexpensive. Influenza is at the opposite extreme. The disease changes slightly from year to year,

---

money implies that life and health have no value. Since they clearly do have value, the way to evaluate prevention, as anything else, is to look at all the costs and benefits and ask whether the benefits are great enough to warrant the costs.

98. Hinman and others, "Progress in Measles Elimination."

and a major change occurs every ten years or so, with the result that old vaccines and old immunities are no longer protective. The vaccine must constantly be reformulated to combat the new disease, and individuals revaccinated. At the same time, the disease is mild enough in most healthy people, missing many altogether in a given year, that the expense and side effects of frequent vaccination for the general population often do not seem worthwhile. Official recommendations for vaccination against influenza concentrate on high-risk groups—the elderly, for example, for whom even a mild case of flu can be life-threatening.

Rubella poses the issue of choosing populations for a different reason. The disease is mild in most cases. But when pregnant women are infected, rubella often causes serious deformities (congenital rubella syndrome) in their unborn children. When a vaccine became available, the question arose whether to vaccinate young children, thereby preventing both the disease and its consequences for pregnant women; or to vaccinate teenage girls, thereby preventing congenital rubella syndrome by protecting women during their fertile years, while leaving most of the population unprotected against the disease. The United States chose the first strategy, the United Kingdom the second. One analysis has shown that if a very high proportion of young children is vaccinated and the immunity conferred is lifelong, the first strategy not only prevents the disease but is more successful against congenital rubella syndrome. But if the proportion vaccinated falls below about 70 percent, the reservoir of vulnerable people can mean that congenital rubella syndrome runs in cycles, at times rising above the levels that would have occurred without vaccination (since, without it, most women are naturally immune by the time they reach adulthood).[99]

Thus the population appropriate for a preventive measure is not a matter that can be entirely separated from the *risks* associated with the disease and the vaccine. When the risk from the disease is high and fairly evenly spread, and the risk from the vaccine is low, vaccination of the entire population is logical. In other instances, the balance of risks may be quite different from one group to another, or from one time to another. Smallpox is the outstanding example. When the disease was endemic in

99. E. G. Knox, "Strategy for Rubella Vaccination," *International Journal of Epidemiology*, vol. 9, no. 1 (1980), pp. 13–23. Schoenbaum and his colleagues reached similar conclusions. Stephen C. Schoenbaum and others, "Benefit-Cost Analysis of Rubella Vaccination Policy," *New England Journal of Medicine*, vol. 294 (February 5, 1976), pp. 306–10.

the United States, vaccination for everyone seemed well justified, given that the vaccine was reasonably safe. But even as the risk from the vaccine declined because of improved techniques of production and administration, the risk from the disease declined faster, until finally the risk from the vaccine was the greater and routine vaccination was discontinued.

When the risk from the disease is clearly much greater than that from the vaccine, estimates of those risks need not be precise for people to conclude that vaccination is worthwhile. But when the risks are close, or when they converge as conditions change, this *uncertainty* becomes important. Whooping cough vaccine, for example, was not developed until the death rate from whooping cough had already fallen to very low levels, a situation similar to that for measles. The vaccine was well accepted at first, but recent studies suggesting that its risks may be relatively large have aroused distrust and resistance among parents in several European countries—Sweden has officially stopped offering the vaccine. More carefully designed studies, undertaken to resolve the controversy, suggest that though some of the earlier estimates of risks were too high, the vaccine nonetheless does cause acute neurologic conditions—in the range of one disorder for every 44,000 to 360,000 vaccinations.[100]

Reducing the range of uncertainty becomes important under conditions like these, but it is difficult to do. In a review of the early trials of pneumococcal pneumonia vaccine, the Office of Technology Assessment noted that, with any fairly safe vaccine, it is virtually impossible to pinpoint the incidence of serious reactions before the vaccine is made available to the general public.[101] Only in groups as large as the entire population will rare reactions occur in sufficient numbers to be noticed and linked to the vaccine. The studies of side effects from smallpox vaccine undertaken in the 1960s are a case in point. Only eight deaths and a few hundred hospitalizations occurred as the result of 14 million vaccinations each year. A trial involving even tens of thousands of participants might not occasion a single death or other severe reaction.

100. D. L. Miller, R. Alderslade, and E. M. Ross, "Whooping Cough and Whooping Cough Vaccine: The Risks and Benefits Debate," in Neal Nathanson and Leon Gordis, eds., *Epidemiologic Reviews*, vol. 4 (1982), pp. 1–23.
101. Office of Technology Assessment, *A Review of Selected Federal Vaccine and Immunization Policies: Based on Case Studies of Pneumococcal Vaccine* (GPO, 1979), especially pp. 56–60.

Smallpox also illustrates a point made earlier—that it is not terribly important to achieve precise estimates of the risk from a safe vaccine until the risk from the disease falls to quite low levels.

People respond differently to the balance of risks, depending on their *individual values*. Some people prefer the low risk of serious flu to the higher risk of a mild reaction to the flu vaccine, while others prefer the possible side effects of the vaccine to the threat of the disease. Reactions are also influenced by particular circumstances that lead people to believe that their personal risks differ from the average. For example, people are more likely to refuse vaccination for themselves or their children if someone in the family has previously suffered side effects from vaccination.[102]

Time affects the balance of these subjective costs and benefits as well as the more objective ones. Just as future expenditures are given less weight than present ones, future gains in health (avoiding the disease) are discounted relative to present ones (avoiding the vaccination). This is one reason people are more reluctant to accept vaccination when the disease is nowhere to be seen than during an outbreak. In the latter case the benefits are likely to be immediate. In the former, the risks of vaccination are immediate, but the benefits may not be received for years, if ever.

102. Nellie Adjaye, "Measles Immunization: Some Factors Affecting Non-Acceptance of Vaccine," *Public Health,* vol. 95 (July 1981), pp. 185–88.

chapter three **Screening**

The goal of screening is to detect disease in its earliest stages, before the patient is aware of any symptoms, when treatment may be most successful. Screening is less truly preventive than vaccination, since a disease, or a precursor, must be established before it can be applied. In the terminology of public health, screening is secondary prevention, while vaccination is primary prevention.

The requirements for successful screening are correspondingly more complex. First, the disease must have a recognizable early stage, or precursor. Second, there must be a reasonably inexpensive and accurate way to diagnose the early stage. Finally, there must be an effective therapy, one that is more effective when applied early than anything that can be done later when the disease has become obvious.[1]

All these elements came together in the early 1970s to make hypertension, or high blood pressure, the focus of a major new prevention effort. The relation between hypertension and disease had been firmly established through longitudinal studies of initially healthy populations— particularly the Framingham study, which recorded the incidence of cardiovascular disease over more than two decades, beginning in 1950, in a sample of the population of Framingham, Massachusetts. Then in reports published in 1967 and 1970, the Veterans' Administration Cooperative Study Group demonstrated the value of symptomatic treatment—reducing blood pressure by means of drugs—for moderate and severe hypertension. This randomized, controlled trial showed sharply lower death rates in the treated group over just a few years, as well as lower rates of nonfatal disease. The results persuaded the medical community of the importance of treating moderate and severe hypertension, and the National High Blood Pressure Education Program was

1. See, for example, the discussion in David M. Eddy, *Screening for Cancer: Theory, Analysis, and Design* (Prentice-Hall, 1980), overview and chap. 1.

launched by the National Heart Institute in 1972 to spread the word to physicians and patients nationwide.

The VA study did not, however, produce a statistically significant difference between the treated and control groups for patients with mild hypertension. As the educational program went forward during the 1970s, interest and controversy centered on the value of treatment for this group, and for women, since the patients in the VA study were all men. Major clinical trials were undertaken to evaluate drug treatment for mild hypertension, and by the late 1970s and the early 1980s, results had come in from several of these trials. Many interpreted the data as unequivocal support for treating mild hypertension with drugs, but others drew more cautious conclusions. At issue in the debate is the medical care of tens of millions of people.

Natural History of Hypertension

Blood pressure is measured at two points during the heart's cycle of contraction and relaxation. The higher pressure, called the systolic pressure, is taken at the peak of the contraction. The lower, or diastolic, pressure is measured when the heart is relaxed. The readings are reported in millimeters of mercury (mm Hg), and a common, normal reading for an adult is 120/80.

The distributions of the two pressures in the adult population are peaked, with most people between 110 and 160 mm Hg for systolic and 70 and 100 mm Hg for diastolic. There is a rapid drop-off outside those ranges, but a somewhat larger number report high pressures than low pressures. The correlation between the two pressures is close; for example, a person with a high diastolic pressure will almost always have a high systolic pressure as well.[2]

More detailed data show that the distributions of pressures differ by age, sex, and race. The higher pressures are less common among women than men until middle age; at older ages, they occur with about the same frequency. In industrialized societies, blood pressure rises somewhat

---

2. The most common exception occurs in the elderly, who sometimes develop high systolic pressures even though their diastolic pressures remain in the intermediate range. William B. Kannel and others, "Systolic Blood Pressure, Arterial Rigidity, and Risk of Stroke: The Framingham Study," *Journal of the American Medical Association*, vol. 245 (March 27, 1981), pp. 1225–29.

with age.[3] As a result, the distributions for older people are flatter, with fewer in the intermediate range and more at the higher pressures. High pressures are also considerably more common among blacks than whites at every age.

Nobody really knows why people develop hypertension in most cases. More than 90 percent of hypertension is "essential" hypertension, meaning that its cause is unknown.[4] Studies of different human populations and of animals have established strong associations between hypertension and heredity (hypertension runs in families), overweight, and salt, and have suggested an association with stress, but so far no single or dominant factor has been identified.[5] The Framingham study found that people who developed hypertension usually had blood pressures toward the upper end of the range even as young adults. Thus most people eventually diagnosed as hypertensive started out with relatively high pressures and were pushed over the diagnostic line by the modest rise that occurs with age. The rest were people whose pressures, low in youth, rose faster than average for some, usually unknown, reason.

In most people hypertension produces no symptoms for the best part of their lives. Recent research indicates that headaches and other symptoms once thought to be caused by high blood pressure are no more common among hypertensives than among normotensives.[6] In later life, however, people with hypertension suffer a higher-than-average rate of illness and death from cardiovascular conditions—coronary heart dis-

3. Thomas Royle Dawber, *The Framingham Study: The Epidemiology of Atherosclerotic Disease* (Harvard University Press, 1980), chap. 6; and Antoon Amery and others, "Hypertension in the Elderly," *Acta Medica Scandinavica,* vol. 210, no. 3 (1981), pp. 221–29.

4. Hypertension Study Group of the Inter-Society Commission for Heart Disease Resources, "Guidelines for Detection, Diagnosis and Management of Hypertensive Populations," *Circulation,* vol. 64 (November 1981), pp. 1079A–89A; and Norman M. Kaplan, *Clinical Hypertension* (New York: Medcom Press, 1973), p. 47.

5. Dawber, *Framingham Study;* Hypertension Study Group, "Guidelines for Detection"; Joint National Committee on Detection, Evaluation, and Treatment of High Blood Pressure, "The 1980 Report of the Joint National Committee on Detection, Evaluation, and Treatment of High Blood Pressure," *Archives of Internal Medicine,* vol. 140 (October 1980), pp. 1280–85; and Gaddo Onesti and Christian R. Klimt, eds., *Hypertension: Determinants, Complications, and Intervention,* Fifth Hahnemann International Symposium on Hypertension (New York: Grune and Stratton, 1979), pt. 1.

6. Milton C. Weinstein and William B. Stason, *Hypertension: A Policy Perspective* (Harvard University Press, 1976), chap. 1; and Noel S. Weiss, "Relation of High Blood Pressure to Headache, Epistaxis, and Selected Other Symptoms," *New England Journal of Medicine,* vol. 287 (September 28, 1972), pp. 631–33.

ease, stroke, and kidney disease. The association between stroke and hypertension is especially strong.

Many researchers had observed the link between hypertension and disease, particularly cardiovascular disease, before the Framingham study. The aim of that study was to establish the link much more precisely by following the development of cardiovascular disease as it occurred in a population initially free of disease, rather than trying to reconstruct events and their causes after the fact. Both fatal and nonfatal cases of disease were recorded. Although blood pressures were measured repeatedly during the study, those taken at the beginning were used to classify the outcomes for each individual, a true test of blood pressure's role as a precursor.[7]

Over the twenty-four years of observation, people in the study who had hypertension at the outset suffered considerably higher rates of coronary heart disease (angina pectoris, myocardial infarction, coronary insufficiency, and sudden death) and cerebrovascular accident (stroke) than those with low blood pressure (table 3-1). For example, men aged 30 to 39 at the beginning of the study with systolic pressures of 180 or higher were more than four times as likely to develop coronary heart disease as men of the same age with systolic pressures below 120. More generally, the rate of disease rose steadily with the level of pressure—the higher the pressure, the greater the risk. And equal increments in pressure tended to be associated with larger and larger increases in risk.[8]

The data showed consistently lower rates of coronary heart disease for women than for men of the same age and pressure, suggesting that women suffer less from hypertension; but this does not hold true for cerebrovascular disease. Predictably, the incidence of disease is higher for older people than for younger people with the same pressure, probably because the older people have had elevated blood pressures for that much longer.

When the data were arrayed by diastolic pressures, the results were

7. Blood pressures measured a year or two before the event show an even stronger relation between pressure and disease than those taken at the outset, but the similarity of the two analyses led Dawber to conclude that "blood-pressure measurements made in early adulthood are accurate predictors of those taken later in life." See Dawber, *Framingham Study*, p. 99.

8. Weinstein and Stason also noted this tendency in their regression analysis of the Framingham data. See Weinstein and Stason, *Hypertension: A Policy Perspective,* chap. 2.

Table 3-1. The Framingham Study: Rates of Cardiovascular Disease over Twenty-four Years, by Systolic Blood Pressure

Number of cases per 1,000 population

Type of disease, sex, and age[a]	Systolic pressure				
	Under 120	120–139	140–159	160–179	180 or higher
Coronary heart disease					
Men					
30–39	95	157	243	265	444
40–49	200	292	330	230	536
50–59	238	361	381	453	490
Women					
30–39	43	65	103	185	n.a.
40–49	93	132	222	259	314
50–59	108	180	246	325	419
Cerebrovascular accident					
Men					
30–39	0	12	50	40	111
40–49	48	50	77	131	214
50–59	60	76	107	130	268
Women					
30–39	15	17	44	n.a.	200
40–49	21	35	28	83	87
50–59	31	83	120	134	220

Source: Thomas Royle Dawber, *The Framingham Study: The Epidemiology of Atherosclerotic Disease* (Harvard University Press, 1980), figs. 7-5 and 7-15.
n.a. Not available.
a. Age at the beginning of the study.

broadly similar, but the rise in risk was not as consistent or sharp.[9] Dawber suggests that one reason for this is "the greater difficulty in determining the diastolic pressure precisely because of the narrower range of pressure. When a measurement cannot be readily reproduced, some misclassification is bound to occur."[10] The point is particularly interesting in light of the medical community's emphasis on the diastolic pressure for diagnosis and for setting therapeutic goals.

Since the Framingham study considered only cardiovascular disease, it did not by itself establish that hypertension leads to higher overall disease and death rates—people with normal blood pressures might suffer from other diseases in greater numbers. This point is important in studying the impact of a condition, or a proposed treatment for the condition. A condition that leads to one form of disease may protect

9. Dawber, *Framingham Study*, figs. 7-10 and 7-17.
10. Ibid., p. 105.

Table 3-2. The New Build and Blood Pressure Study: Relative Death Rates,ᵃ by Blood
Pressure, 1954–73

Systolic pressure	Men (percent)	Women (percent)	Diastolic pressure	Men (percent)	Women (percent)
88–97	70	92	48–67	84	87
98–127	85	91	68–82	94	97
128–137	111	108	83–87	119	115
138–147	136	122	88–92	138	133
148–157	168	135	93–97	171	163
158–167	210	167	98–102	204	183
168–177	224	n.a.			
178–192	232	n.a.			

Source: Edward Lew, "The New Build and Blood Pressure Study," *Transactions of the Association of Life Insurance Medical Directors of America,* vol. 62 (1978), p. 164.
n.a. Not available.
a. Percentages of the rate of people with pressures of about 120 (systolic) and 80 (diastolic). Source does not specify when the blood pressure measurements were taken.

against another, and a treatment that reduces one form of disease may cause another. Only data on total mortality and disease can show whether the net result is a gain or a loss.

One of the early studies to establish the link between hypertension and total death rates was the 1959 Build and Blood Pressure Study, carried out by the life insurance industry and updated in 1978.[11] The New Build and Blood Pressure Study, as it was called, was based on 4.5 million insured people, whose records were followed in many cases for more than twenty years, from the early 1950s to the early 1970s. This population was somewhat healthier and wealthier than the national population, and people over 50 had somewhat lower blood pressures than the national average in both the 1959 and the new studies.

In the new study the death rates for men with systolic pressures above 157 were about double or more than double those for men with pressures below 138 (table 3-2). A similar picture emerges from the data arranged by diastolic pressure. For women, higher blood pressure is also associated with higher mortality, but the rise is considerably less steep. Again, it appears that hypertension is less detrimental for women; this is reflected in the view of some practitioners that the diagnostic dividing line should be set higher for women than for men.[12] Comparison of these results with those from the 1959 study show that death rates were lower

11. Edward Lew, "The New Build and Blood Pressure Study," *Transactions of the Association of Life Insurance Medical Directors of America,* vol. 62 (1978), pp. 154–74.

12. Kaplan, *Clinical Hypertension,* pp. 3, 5–9.

for men at all blood pressures in the new study, and lower for women at the high end of the pressure range.[13] Presumably the shift reflects improvements in health and in medical care unrelated to hypertension.

The relation between blood pressure and cardiovascular disease is a statistical relation, true on average for a population but not necessarily true for each individual in the population. Some people never suffer any ill effects from their hypertension. Unfortunately, there is no known way to distinguish those in which hypertension is, or will prove to be, benign, from those in which it will eventually produce complications.[14]

How Many People Have Hypertension?

There is no natural dividing line between normal and high blood pressure. As described in the last section, studies have consistently shown that the higher the pressure, the higher the risk of illness and death. But arbitrary lines have been drawn for the practical purpose of deciding whether treatment is worthwhile and for classifying the severity of risk involved. In its 1971–75 and 1976–80 surveys, the National Center for Health Statistics followed standard practice in specifying definite hypertension as a systolic pressure of 160 mm Hg or higher, a diastolic pressure of 95 mm Hg or higher, or both. Normotension was defined as pressures below 140/90, and everything in between was labeled borderline hypertension.[15] These are consistent with the World Health Organization's definition of hypertension as pressures of 160 and/or 95 or higher.[16] Although the Framingham study showed that systolic pressures are better predictors of risk, some definitions use only the diastolic pressure, especially the division of hypertension into mild (90–104), moderate (105–114), and severe (115 or higher) used in the classic Veterans' Administration study. The same or closely similar dividing lines have been used in other studies and in many policy statements.[17]

Based on blood pressure measurements taken during a single examination, a large proportion of the adult population has some degree of

13. Lew, "New Build and Blood Pressure Study," p. 164.
14. Kaplan, *Clinical Hypertension,* p. 67.
15. See, for example, National Center for Health Statistics, *Hypertension in Adults 25–74 Years of Age, United States, 1971–1975,* Vital Health Statistics Series 11, no. 221 (Hyattsville, Md.: Department of Health and Human Services, 1981), p. 11.
16. Amery and others, "Hypertension in the Elderly," p. 221.
17. Joint National Committee, "1980 Report," p. 1281.

Figure 3-1. Distributions of Natural Blood Pressures in the U.S. Population, 1980

Millions of people

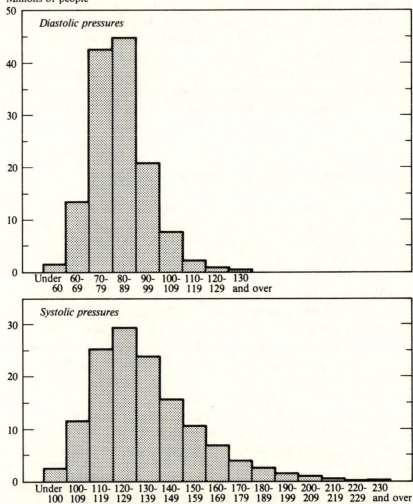

Sources: Author's calculations based on data from National Center for Health Statistics, *Hypertension in Adults 25–74 Years of Age, United States, 1971–1975*, Vital Health Statistics Series 11, no. 221 (Hyattsville, Md.: Department of Health and Human Services, 1981), tables 2–11; and population data from Bureau of the Census, *Census of Population, 1980*, Supplementary Report PC80-S1-1, "Age, Sex, Race, and Spanish Origin of the Population by Regions, Divisions, and States: 1980" (Government Printing Office, 1981), p. 3.

hypertension. Figure 3-1 presents estimates of the distributions of naturally occurring pressures, that is, those that would be observed if no one with hypertension were treated, for 1980. It shows that an estimated 10 million adults 25 or older had diastolic pressures of 100 or more. An additional 21 million people had pressures between 90 and

100—a huge number that underscores the importance of the debate over treating mild hypertension.[18]

For diagnosis and treatment, however, a single measurement, or even several measurements during a single visit, is not enough. An individual's pressures fluctuate with the time of day, level of activity, stress, and other factors. Thus before treatment is undertaken, it is important to be sure that the individual's pressures are consistently elevated and not simply the result of some temporary circumstance.[19]

Several statistical studies have considered how many visits and how many pressure readings per visit are necessary to be reasonably sure of identifying a person as hypertensive, that is, as having consistently elevated pressures.[20] One analysis concludes that a reasonable and practicable choice—balancing the gains from greater reliability against the costs in time and money of the additional visits—is to take at least two measurements during each of three separate visits. This standard is recommended in its 1980 and 1984 reports by the Joint National Committee on Detection, Evaluation, and Treatment of High Blood Pressure, which notes that "after screening, the diagnosis of hypertension is confirmed when the average of multiple BP [blood pressure] measurements made on at least two subsequent visits is 90 mm Hg or higher."[21]

18. The estimates were derived by applying the distributions of blood pressure by age and sex recorded for a national sample during the years 1971–75 to the population by age and sex in 1980. Drug treatment of hypertension was much less common in the early 1970s than it is now, and even when prescribed, it was often not pursued vigorously enough to bring the patient's pressure down to the normal range. (See Hypertension Study Group, "Guidelines for Detection," p. 1080A.) Thus figure 3-1 is a reasonable approximation to the naturally occurring distributions of pressures in the adult population.

19. The underlying assumption—an entirely reasonable one—is that people with consistently elevated pressures are at greatest risk. Presumably, had the Framingham study identified those with consistently high pressures at the beginning, rather than those with a single high reading, the study would have shown an even stronger relation between pressure and risk.

20. For example, see Bernard Rosner and B. Frank Polk, "The Implications of Blood Pressure Variability for Clinical and Screening Purposes," *Journal of Chronic Diseases*, vol. 32, no. 6 (1979), pp. 451–61; and Donald S. Shepard, "Reliability of Blood Pressure Measurements: Implications for Designing and Evaluating Programs to Control Hypertension," *Journal of Chronic Diseases*, vol. 34, no. 5 (1981), pp. 191–209.

21. Joint National Committee, "1980 Report," p. 1280, and "The 1984 Report of the Joint National Committee on Detection, Evaluation, and Treatment of High Blood Pressure," *Archives of Internal Medicine*, vol. 14 (March 1984), p. 1045. A Canadian group recommends at least three retests for persons with diastolic pressures of 90 to 104 and no organ or vessel damage. See Canadian Hypertension Society, *Report of the*

The clinical trials of drug therapy discussed in more detail below confirm the unreliability of single measurements. In the Hypertension Detection and Follow-up Program conducted in the United States by a division of the National Institutes of Health, for example, of about 17,500 people whose diastolic pressures had been 95 or higher at an initial screening, only 63 percent measured 90 or above at a second examination; even though the cutoff point was reduced for the second screening, more than a third of the group fell below it.[22] Similarly, in a study in Oslo, Norway, almost half (46 percent) of the men whose systolic pressures had been 150 or higher at the initial screening fell below this level at two subsequent examinations and were not included in the trial.[23]

The explanation is believed to be that people's pressures are higher at an initial screening because they are anxious about the procedure, and that their pressures drop as they become more familiar with it. Whatever the reason, the problem persists over long periods of time. In a major Australian trial, participants were accepted into the trial if readings taken on two separate occasions showed their diastolic pressure to lie between 95 and 110 and their systolic pressure to lie below 200.[24] Drug treatment (placebo tablets for the control group) was started on the third visit, or as soon thereafter as the individual's diastolic pressure again measured 95 or higher (or the systolic pressure measured 200 or higher). Over an average of four years in the study, 12.8 percent of those accepted as participants on the basis of the first two examinations never again had pressures high enough to warrant treatment; these people were eliminated from the final results.[25]

Such substantial declines from one test to the next indicate that the

Consensus Development Conference on the Management of Mild Hypertension in Canada (Toronto: The Society, 1984), pp. 1–8.

22. Hypertension Detection and Follow-up Program Cooperative Group, "Five-Year Findings of the Hypertension Detection and Follow-up Program: Reduction in Mortality of Persons with High Blood Pressure, Including Mild Hypertension," *Journal of the American Medical Association*, vol. 242 (December 7, 1979), pp. 2562–71.

23. Anders Helgeland, "Treatment of Mild Hypertension—A Five Year Controlled Drug Trial: The Oslo Study," *American Journal of Medicine,* vol. 69 (November 1980), p. 726.

24. Both limits were necessary to be sure that only people with mild hypertension were accepted, while those with moderate or severe hypertension were referred for drug treatment immediately.

25. Management Committee, "The Australian Therapeutic Trial in Mild Hypertension," *The Lancet* (June 14, 1980), pp. 1261–67; and Norman M. Kaplan, "Whom to Treat: The Dilemma of Mild Hypertension," *American Heart Journal*, vol. 101 (June 1981), p. 868.

number of people who would be confirmed as hypertensive after several examinations would be much lower than the numbers derived from figure 3-1. That figure is based on a survey in which each participant's pressures were measured three times during a single examination. Probably the 10 million adults with initial diastolic pressures of 100 or more would continue to fall above 90, but perhaps only half of those with initial readings between 90 and 100 would. Thus the 31 million people with elevated pressures at a first reading might produce just over 20 million with consistently elevated pressures. The Hypertension Study Group of the Inter-Society Commission for Heart Disease Resources acknowledged the problem of attrition, but noted that this still left a huge number of people who posed an "immense challenge" for the medical care system.[26]

Like repeated blood pressure measurements, the diagnostic workup recommended for any patient whose pressures appear to be consistently elevated also helps reduce the risk of misdiagnosis.[27] This workup includes lab tests, a physical exam to discover any hypertensive complications, such as changes in the functioning of the heart or in the pattern of blood vessels in the eye, and a history to find out whether the patient has a family background of hypertension, or habits such as smoking that might put him or her at greater risk for certain diseases. If the patient's pressures are relatively low, no complications have appeared, and there are no other risk factors, the physician may decide to wait and watch. Annual or biannual blood pressure measurements are recommended even for those with normal pressures. As one clinician notes, for each patient, the question must be: when do "investigation and treatment do more good than harm"?[28]

Treatment: The Clinical Trials

Since the success of the Veterans' Administration trials, long-term treatment with antihypertensive drugs has been widely considered the most effective remedy for moderate and severe hypertension. It was unequivocally endorsed, for example, by the Joint National Committee

26. Hypertension Study Group, "Guidelines for Detection," p. 1080A.
27. Ibid.; and Joint National Committee, "1980 Report."
28. Kaplan, *Clinical Hypertension,* p. 7, quoting J. G. Evans and G. Rose, *British Medical Bulletin,* vol. 27 (1971).

on High Blood Pressure in its 1980 and 1984 reports.[29] The committee recommended that therapy proceed in steps, beginning with a diuretic and adding larger doses and different types of drugs (adrenergic inhibiting agents and vasodilators) until the patient's diastolic pressure drops below 90. Diuretics, which reduce blood volume and the level of sodium in the blood by increasing the excretion of urine, are safest and sufficient for many people. Often, however, experimentation with drugs and dosages is necessary not only to reduce blood pressure but to minimize side effects, and the committee granted that if side effects remained a problem, the physician might have to be satisfied with a diastolic pressure somewhat higher than 90. Weight control and reduction of salt in the diet were recommended as adjuncts to drug therapy, because they have some independent effect in reducing blood pressures and thus may permit smaller doses of drugs, and because they help control side effects.

Although the VA trials had generated great excitement over the potential of drug treatment, they had been too small and too short to show whether drugs helped people with mild hypertension. Plans were laid almost as soon as their results were published to field new trials to answer this question. Compared with most clinical trials, these studies were huge. The Oslo, Norway, trial involved 785 men aged 40 to 49; the Australian trial, 3,427 men and women 30 to 69; the U.S. Hypertension Detection and Follow-up Program, 10,940 men and women 30 to 69. The trials were necessarily lengthy and results did not begin to appear until 1979.[30]

The U.S. Hypertension Detection and Follow-up Program accepted everyone in 14 communities whose diastolic pressure averaged 90 or above over three visits. Since the planning committee decided that it would be unethical to deny treatment to anyone, the study had no control group. Instead, the participants were randomly assigned either to care in special clinics or to a doctor in the community (the "referred" group);

29. Joint National Committee, "1980 Report," pp. 1281–83, and "1984 Report," pp. 1047–53.

30. The largest of all—the United Kingdom's Medical Research Council trial, which aimed to include 18,000 men and women 35 to 64—was scheduled to be completed in August 1985. W. E. Miall and P. J. Brennan, "The Financial Implications and Feasibility of a National Multicentre Therapeutic Trial for Mild Hypertension in the United Kingdom," in Onesti and Klimt, eds., *Hypertension*, pp. 373–80; Medical Research Council Working Party on Mild to Moderate Hypertension, "Adverse Reactions to Bendrofluazide and Propranolol for the Treatment of Mild Hypertension," *The Lancet* (September 12, 1981), pp. 539–43; and Canadian Hypertension Society, *Report of the Consensus Development Conference*, pp. 2–19.

the study staff tried to ensure that everyone in the referred group with a diastolic pressure of 115 or higher, or hypertensive complications, actually did see a doctor. Those in the clinic group were given drugs according to a stepped regimen like that endorsed by the Joint National Committee on High Blood Pressure. Exactly what treatment was prescribed for the referred group is not known, although the study did record whether these patients received antihypertensive drugs.[31]

Thus the trial was a comparison of more vigorous with less vigorous care, rather than a comparison of drug treatment with no treatment. After five years, mortality in the clinic group was significantly less than mortality in the referred group—6.4 per 100 persons compared with 7.7 per 100. Of particular interest, the difference was just as large for those with mild hypertension (about 70 percent of the participants)—5.9 per 100 compared with 7.4 per 100. There is no way to know, of course, how either group would have compared with a group of untreated hypertensives, and even the apparent meaning of the results is muddied by the fact that there were fewer deaths in the clinic group from causes unrelated to hypertension as well as from related causes. One observer has suggested that the result may have been partly due to the more careful medical attention received by the clinic patients rather than to treatment for hypertension specifically.[32]

The Oslo and Australian trials included only mild hypertensives with no signs of complications—a large proportion of the hypertensive population. In the Oslo trial, men were randomly assigned to receive drug treatment or no treatment for five years. The Australian trial randomly assigned participants to receive active drugs or placebos; the length of time depended on when the participant entered the trial, averaging between three and four years. All participants in this trial were examined regularly by the study staff, thus eliminating the possibility that differences in medical attention might affect the outcome.[33]

In both trials, participants in the control groups whose pressures rose above certain limits (180/110 in the Oslo trial, 200/110 in the Australian trial) were given drugs. Thus the trials compared aggressive treatment with a more conservative approach in which the patient was followed

31. Hypertension Detection and Follow-up Group, "Five-Year Findings," pp. 2563–64.

32. Kaplan, "Whom to Treat," p. 867.

33. Helgeland, "Treatment of Mild Hypertension," pp. 725–32; and Management Committee, "Australian Therapeutic Trial."

but drugs were withheld unless and until the patient's pressures rose into the moderate range. This comparison is particularly useful because, in practice, the choice between aggressive and conservative management of mild, uncomplicated hypertension is probably the one that concerns doctors and patients most. When the lifelong drug treatment of millions of people is at issue, the possibility of postponing treatment for several years, or even much longer, is important.

Looking at the participants as a group, the author of the Oslo report concluded that "neither total mortality nor mortality from cardiovascular events was influenced by drug treatment."[34] Although hypertensive complications and cerebrovascular deaths occurred only in the control group, coronary events were somewhat more frequent in the treated group. The Australian trial, on the other hand, found that the death rate from all causes was significantly lower for the treated group—1.7 per 1,000 person-years compared with 3.7. The rate of nonfatal cardiovascular events was also lower.

One expert on the subject has suggested that closer examination of both trials supports a somewhat different and more consistent conclusion, namely, that drug treatment did not help participants whose diastolic pressures averaged less than 100 during the trial.[35] The Oslo report noted that those with diastolic pressures consistently above 100 suffered fewer cardiovascular events if they were receiving drug treatment. The Australian report shows that those in the placebo group whose diastolic pressures averaged less than 100 during the trial had fewer deaths and cardiovascular events than those whose pressures were reduced to the same level with the help of medication.[36] This might mean only that an artificially lowered pressure is not as beneficial as a natural pressure of the same level, but it raises the possibility that there are no net benefits from drug therapy for the group with pressures under 100.[37] The point is important, since 80 percent of the placebo group had diastolic pressures below 100 throughout the trial (although half had had readings above 100 at the initial screening). The expert concludes that

34. Helgeland, "Treatment of Mild Hypertension," p. 728.
35. Kaplan, "Whom to Treat," p. 867.
36. Helgeland, "Treatment of Mild Hypertension," p. 730; and Management Committee, "Australian Therapeutic Trial," table 10.
37. A noteworthy exception is the large group in the Australian trial whose diastolic pressures at the initial screening were 95–99. Those whose pressures were reduced below 90 by medication had a lower rate of death and illness than those whose pressures fell below 90 naturally.

"drug therapy for *uncomplicated* hypertension is indicated only for those whose diastolic blood pressures remain at or above 100 mm Hg after 6 months of nondrug therapy."[38]

Two major reasons for so much caution in concluding that drugs help mild hypertension are the cost of treatment, discussed below, and the side effects. To the extent that objective side effects manifest themselves as disease, and not just as abnormal test results, they are taken into account in trials with untreated control groups. When the treated hypertensives suffer fewer deaths and illnesses, it is correct to conclude that the beneficial effects of medication on these outcomes outweigh any adverse effects. Measures of illness and death do not, however, reflect the so-called subjective side effects, such as fatigue or depression. For example, the Oslo study questioned participants after four years, when drug regimens were stable, and found that fatigue, drowsiness, impotence, and gout were more common in the treated group. Since untreated hypertension is usually asymptomatic, effects like these lead many patients to discontinue therapy.

Some side effects, especially worry, may arise as much from the fact of diagnosis as from any treatment. In a health insurance experiment conducted by the Rand Corporation, people who reported having been diagnosed as hypertensive, though found not to be on examination, reported worry or pain much more frequently than did others with normal pressures. People with a confirmed diagnosis of hypertension were even more likely to report some worry or pain.[39] Within this group, those on medication reported pain or worry more often than those not on it. The authors of the Rand report suggest that those on drugs may have had more severe hypertension, although the differences remain even when borderline hypertensives (140/90–159/94) and definite hypertensives (160/95 or higher) are considered separately. In a similar vein, a Canadian study found that absenteeism increased sharply among hypertensive steelworkers after their hypertension was diagnosed.[40] Both studies suggest that there are harmful side effects simply to labeling people hypertensive.

38. Kaplan, "Whom to Treat," p. 867.
39. Robert H. Brook and others, *Conceptualization and Measurement of Physiologic Health for Adults*, vol. 3: *Hypertension*, Rand Health Insurance Experiment Series R-2262/3-HHS (Santa Monica, Calif.: Rand Corp., August 1980), pp. 32, 34.
40. Canadian Hypertension Society, *Report of the Consensus Development Conference*, chap. 3.

None of the available trials has tracked participants for longer than five years. This cutoff point has two important implications. Since the advantages of treatment have shown up more quickly the more severe the hypertension, trials of only a few years may not be sufficient to indicate whether aggressive drug treatment is beneficial for mild hypertension over the long run. Second, for all degrees of hypertension, the trials are not long enough to provide solid information about the benefits and risks of truly long-term drug treatment. Some of them show the advantage of the treated group growing larger over the few years of the study, and this pattern may continue indefinitely. Or the detrimental effects of drugs may begin to outweigh the benefits as time passes. With so many people on drug treatment, it is important to know which is the case.

There are alternatives to drug therapy. A number of studies indicate that losing weight and reducing dietary salt can lower blood pressures. Averaging over several studies, one review reported that systolic pressures dropped 3 points and diastolic pressures 2 points for every kilogram (2.2 pounds) of weight lost, up to 10 kilograms;[41] a patient who lost 10 kilograms might thereby reduce his or her pressures by 30/20 points, on average, a substantial reduction and one sufficient to bring many people into the normal range. The same review reported that a decline in salt intake from 12 grams (about 6 teaspoons) to 6 grams a day reduced the pressures by 11 and 10 points, on average. American adults are estimated to consume 4 to 5 grams of salt a day, an amount considered excessive by many experts.[42] The joint effect of simultaneously reducing weight and salt is not known.

Recent studies have produced evidence that the amount and kinds of fat in the diet may have a strong effect on blood pressure. A study conducted in Finland found that people put on diets low in fat, particularly saturated fats, experienced a substantial drop in blood pressure over only six weeks, although they did not lose weight.[43] Those in the control group and, interestingly, those put on a low-salt diet, showed no change in blood pressure during the study. An Australian study that experimented with a vegetarian diet, which contains substantially less saturated

41. A. Amery and others, "Does Diet Matter in Hypertension?" *European Heart Journal*, vol. 1 (August 1980), pp. 299–308.

42. "Salt: A New Villain?" *Time* (March 15, 1982), p. 64.

43. Pekka Puska and others, "Controlled, Randomized Trial of the Effect of Dietary Fat on Blood Pressure," *The Lancet* (January 1/8, 1983), pp. 1–9.

fat than the more usual diet, also reported that it led to a drop in participants' blood pressures.[44]

Nothing like the resources expended on trials of drug therapy have been committed to testing these alternatives. Studies of them are invariably small, usually short-term, and often poorly controlled. One of the largest and best of the studies of weight control involved 107 patients, only 24 of them treated by diet alone, and followed them for only seven months.[45] Another study carefully compared salt restriction with no treatment and with two different drug regimens, but had only 31 patients in each of the four groups.[46] Probably because of their small scale, these studies have focused on the intermediate goal of therapy, lowering blood pressure, rather than the ultimate goal, reductions in illness and deaths. Although lower pressures are associated with less disease and death, and both interventions are assumed to be without important risks, the definitive tests of these assumptions are rates of disease and death.

Current Status of the Debate

Efforts during the last decade to educate physicians and the public about the importance of treating hypertension have paid off. National surveys show that, in 1976–80, three-quarters of those found during the survey examination to have a systolic pressure of at least 160, a diastolic pressure of at least 95, or both, had already been diagnosed as hypertensive, compared with only half in 1960–62 and just under two-thirds in 1974–75.[47] More than half were taking medication, compared with about a third in the two earlier periods. The proportion whose pressures had been reduced below 160/95 by medication was also much higher in the 1976–80 period—34 percent compared with 16 percent in 1960–62 and

44. Ian L. Rouse and others, "Blood-Pressure-Lowering Effect of a Vegetarian Diet: Controlled Trial in Normotensive Subjects," *The Lancet* (January 1/8, 1983), pp. 5–9.

45. Efrain Reisin and others, "Effect of Weight Loss without Salt Restriction on the Reduction of Blood Pressure in Overweight Hypertensive Patients," *New England Journal of Medicine*, vol. 298 (January 5, 1978), pp. 1–6.

46. T. Morgan and others, "Hypertension Treated by Salt Restriction," *The Lancet* (February 4, 1978), pp. 227–30.

47. Michael Rowland and Jean Roberts, "Blood Pressure Levels and Hypertension in Persons Ages 6–74 Years: United States, 1976–80," *National Center for Health Statistics Advance Data*, no. 84 (October 8, 1982), table 7.

58   Is Prevention Better Than Cure?

20 percent in 1974–75. Many people believe these trends have contributed to the sharp decline in deaths from stroke since 1972.[48]

The remaining gaps in treatment reflect several factors. Not everyone with pressures over 160/95 at a single examination proves to have consistently elevated pressure. And for those who do, the side effects of medication may make it undesirable to reduce the pressure to the normal range. But the gaps also reflect the continuing debate over the treatment appropriate for patients with mild hypertension, particularly those with diastolic pressures between 90 and 100.

The Joint National Committee on High Blood Pressure published its first recommendations in 1980, a year after the results of the Hypertension Detection and Follow-up Program were first reported. As noted above, the committee advocated drug treatment for people with moderate or severe hypertension without qualification. Its advice for patients with mild hypertension was more guarded. The committee suggested that nondrug therapy, principally weight reduction and salt restriction, be tried first, a suggestion later endorsed by the Hypertension Study Group of the Inter-Society Commission for Heart Disease Resources in its 1981 report.[49] "If diet proves ineffective in normalizing BP [blood pressure] after an adequate trial," the committee continued, "drug therapy should be considered in addition."[50] The decision to use drugs for patients with mild hypertension depends not only on the levels of pressure, but on whether there is evidence of hypertensive complications or other factors (smoking, family history) associated with higher mortality. The committee granted that in young patients without complications, the side effects and costs of long-term drug treatment might not outweigh the benefits.

Meanwhile, because of the uncertainty in the medical community about the implications of their results for mild hypertension, the investigators of the Hypertension Detection and Follow-up Program published a more detailed analysis in 1982.[51] As already described, the trial compared an aggressive regimen of medication for patients treated in the study's clinics with the unknown but presumably less aggressive

48. "Incidence of Strokes Declines," *Science*, vol. 220 (May 6, 1983), p. 591.
49. Joint National Committee, "1980 Report," p. 1282; and Hypertension Study Group, "Guidelines for Detection," p. 1082A.
50. Joint National Committee, "1980 Report," p. 1282.
51. Hypertension Detection and Follow-up Program Cooperative Group, "The Effect of Treatment on Mortality in 'Mild' Hypertension: Results of the Hypertension Detection and Follow-up Program," *New England Journal of Medicine*, vol. 307 (October 14, 1982), pp. 976–80.

care given those who were referred to their doctors after screening. The goal for each patient in the clinic group whose diastolic pressure was between 90 and 100 was to reduce it by 10 points. Given the state of knowledge at the time of the trial, the patients referred to their physicians were much less likely to have received medication or to have been treated aggressively if they did receive it.

The investigators showed that, no matter how the participants with mild hypertension were subdivided, those treated in the clinics had lower mortality rates than those referred to their physicians. They examined the outcomes separately for participants with diastolic pressures of 90–94, 95–99, and 100–104. They separated out those who had no hypertensive complications and were not already on drugs when they joined the study and looked at the same three groups again. In every case, mortality was lower for those treated in the clinics. The investigators granted that factors other than drug treatment alone, such as the close supervision and free medication given the clinic patients, might have played a part in the outcome, but they nonetheless concluded that the results supported a recommendation that drug treatment be considered early for those with mild hypertension.

Guidelines subsequently published by an expert group convened by the World Health Organization and the International Society of Hypertension edged closer to recommending that patients with mild hypertension routinely receive medication. The assembled experts proposed a careful protocol based on repeated testing of people with diastolic pressures above 90. Medication was urged at once for those whose pressures remained over 100 for a month. General health measures and further observation were recommended for those with lower pressures, followed by medication for any whose pressures remained above 95 after three more months of observation. The experts noted that in some cases side effects might prevent reducing pressure below 90, the goal, and that they were an especially important consideration for mild hypertension, since "the individual benefits to be expected from treatment are not very large."[52] Nonetheless, for the first time people with diastolic pressures between 95 and 100 were counted among those for whom drugs were the treatment of choice.

In its 1984 report, the Joint National Committee on High Blood Pressure took a still stronger line, counseling drug therapy for anyone

52. "Guidelines for the Treatment of Mild Hypertension: Memorandum from a W.H.O./I.S.H. Meeting," *The Lancet* (February 26, 1983), pp. 457–58.

with a diastolic pressure above 95 and for those with a pressure in the 90–94 range if there was evidence of organ damage or other risk factors.[53] The committee recommended nondrug therapies be tried at first for others in the 90–94 range and granted that drugs remained controversial for this group even when the nondrug measures failed. The Canadian Hypertension Society published similar recommendations in 1984—with the difference that the society still argued that drug treatment should be discretionary for those with diastolic pressures of 95–99 and no organ damage.[54]

The weight of the evidence in favor of drug treatment is already so great in the view of many people that it may be difficult ever to do a proper trial of such alternative therapies as weight and salt control, especially in this country where, before the completion of any major trials of drug treatment for mild hypertension, the designers of the Hypertension Detection and Follow-up Program decided it would be unethical to withhold drugs. Yet the Oslo and Australian trials imply it may not be unethical. The value of drugs for people with diastolic pressures below 100 has not been confirmed by all the major trials. Thus it should be possible to test alternative therapies on mild hypertensives, using the same study design as the Oslo and Australian trials; participants whose pressures rose into the moderate range would be put on drugs. If these alternatives proved their worth for mild hypertensives, it might then be considered ethical to try them on people with somewhat higher pressures.

Both the Joint National Committee on High Blood Pressure (in its 1980 report) and the Hypertension Study Group noted the importance of undertaking larger, better controlled trials of these therapies. According to the Hypertension Study Group, "It is absolutely essential that definitive studies in primary prevention be undertaken involving the control of obesity and sodium intake."[55] Several years earlier, a researcher had recommended a long-term trial of salt restriction beginning in childhood.[56] Various approaches to stress management, such as relaxation therapy, have also been proposed as worthy of more careful

53. Joint National Committee, "1984 Report," pp. 1048–51.

54. Canadian Hypertension Society, *Report of the Consensus Development Conference*, pp. 1–7.

55. Hypertension Study Group, "Guidelines for Detection," p. 1081A.

56. Lot B. Page, "Salt and Hypertension: Epidemiology and Mechanisms," in Onesti and Klimt, eds., *Hypertension*, pp. 3–11.

study.[57] Again, the belief that these approaches are safer and more truly preventive than drug therapy underlies their attractiveness.

More on the Accuracy of Diagnostic Tests

The difficulty of determining who has hypertension illustrates the central problem for all diagnostic tests—how to identify correctly those who have the condition and avoid misdiagnosing those who do not. Conceptually at least, the problem can be divided into two components. One is the reliability of the test as a way of identifying the precursor condition (how accurately does a single measurement reflect the person's usual blood pressure?). The second is the validity of the precursor condition itself as an indicator of the more serious condition that is to be prevented (how strong is the connection between blood pressure and heart disease, kidney disease, and stroke?).[58]

The first element has been a chief concern in hypertension—how accurately single or repeated measurements reflect the person's usual blood pressure. For the Pap smear, interest has focused on the second element as well—how accurately the condition revealed by the test predicts the incidence of cancer of the cervix.[59] Screening aims to identify a precursor of disease, or an initial stage, in the hope that early intervention can prevent the more serious stage from developing. In many cases, however, the precursor or early stage does not proceed inevitably to the full-scale disease. Not everyone with hypertension develops heart disease, kidney disease, or stroke, and not every woman with cervical dysplasia, or even carcinoma in situ, develops invasive

57. Alan P. Brauer and others, "Relaxation Therapy for Essential Hypertension: A Veterans Administration Outpatient Study," *Journal of Behavioral Medicine*, vol. 2 (March 1979), pp. 21–29; and Redford B. Williams, Jr., "Behavioral Approaches in the Prevention and Treatment of Hypertension," in Delores L. Parron, Fredric Solomon, and Robert J. Haggerty, eds., *Combining Psychosocial and Drug Therapy: Hypertension, Depression, and Diabetes* (Washington, D.C.: National Academy Press, 1981), pp. 59–66.

58. This distinction is brought out by A. L. Cochrane, P. A. Graham, and J. Wallace in their paper "Glaucoma," in *Screening in Medical Care: Reviewing the Evidence, A Collection of Essays*, prepared for the Nuffield Provincial Hospitals Trust (Oxford University Press, 1968), pp. 81–88.

59. Anne-Marie Foltz and Jennifer L. Kelsey, "The Annual Pap Test: A Dubious Policy Success," *Milbank Memorial Fund Quarterly/Health and Society*, vol. 56 (Fall 1978), pp. 426–62.

cancer of the cervix. Indeed, rather than progressing, the intermediate condition sometimes spontaneously disappears.

In practice, it can be difficult to separate the two elements. When a Pap smear is positive, but cervical cancer does not develop, is the problem that a Pap smear is an imperfect indicator of dysplasia, or that dysplasia is an imperfect predictor of cervical cancer? There is no direct way to determine how well a test identifies the early stage of a disease. Its accuracy can only be checked by comparing it with another test for the same condition, which is not perfect either, or by waiting to see what course the disease follows. In the latter case, incomplete knowledge of the natural course of the disease can be difficult to distinguish from an inaccurate measure of the precursor condition.[60]

The statistics conventionally used to describe the problem—the sensitivity and specificity of a test—do not attempt to separate out the two components. The *sensitivity* of a test, also called the true-positive rate, is the percentage of those with the condition who show an abnormal, or "positive," test result.[61] The numerator is people with the condition who have positive tests and the denominator is all people with the condition who took the test. Because there is no perfect test, the denominator—those with the condition—cannot be identified with complete accuracy. The *specificity* of the test, also called the true-negative rate, is the percentage of those without the condition who show a normal, or "negative," test result. Especially with continuously distributed variables like blood pressure, the sensitivity of the test generally improves as its specificity declines, and vice versa—it is impossible to improve both at the same time.[62]

The relative importance of sensitivity and specificity rates depends

60. See Eddy, *Screening for Cancer*, especially chap. 4.
61. See Judith S. Mausner and Anita K. Bahn, *Epidemiology: An Introductory Text* (W.B. Saunders Co., 1974), chap. 11.
62. The complements of these two rates are the false-negative rate (those with the condition who are incorrectly identified as normal by the test) and the false-positive rate (those without the condition who are incorrectly identified as having it). In any particular case, all four rates will depend not only on the accuracy of the test but on the characteristics of the patient, the quality of the lab work, and the skill of the practitioner.
To see why sensitivity improves as specificity declines, think of the two groups of people—those with the condition and those without—as being represented by two overlapping bell-shaped curves. Because of the overlap, a cutoff point for diagnosis that picks up more of those with the condition by including more of their curve will also pick up more of those *without* the condition (in the overlapping tail of *their* curve).

critically on the prevalence of the condition. Consider a simple example in which a condition affects 2 of every 1,000 people and the relevant test correctly identifies everyone with the condition (its sensitivity is 100 percent), but 2 percent of people without the condition also test positive (its specificity is 98 percent); this would be an extremely accurate test. Of every 1,000 people tested, 2 will have the condition and will be correctly identified by the test. But about 20 (998 × .02) normal people will also produce positive test results (that is, false positives). Thus 22 people will proceed to the next stage—either further testing to try to confirm the initial diagnosis, or treatment. This may involve unnecessary risk and discomfort for the 20 misdiagnosed people and can be costly; consequently screening can be quite expensive per unit of health benefit, even when the cost per test is low.

The situation looks quite different for a condition that is widespread. Suppose the prevalence of the condition is 100 per 1,000, as it may be for hypertension, while the other rates in the example stay the same. Then 100 people will be correctly identified as having the condition and 18 normal people (900 × .02) will test false-positive. Nearly as many normal people as before (18 versus 20) are at risk for unnecessary further diagnosis or treatment, but the proportions make the initial test look much more worthwhile. In the second case, 85 percent (100 of 118) of those who test positive actually have the condition and may benefit from effective treatment, while in the first case only 9 percent (2 of 22) of those tested are true positives. Their gains must be weighed against the losses of the misdiagnosed people who are subjected to further testing or to treatment. Such considerations have led the medical community to try to distinguish high-risk groups for testing when the prevalence of a condition is low in the general population.

False negatives involve risks of a different sort. A false-negative test result means that the test fails to detect the disease in someone who has it. Thus that person loses the advantages of early detection and treatment. The numbers involved are generally small—with a prevalence of 100 in 1,000, for example, if the sensitivity of the test were 90 percent, "only" 10 people with the disease would be missed. The individual consequences, of course, can be great for someone who could have been spared a serious, even fatal, illness.

Decisions about screening must balance all these elements—the costs of misclassifying patients as well as the benefits and costs of accurately detecting disease in its early stages, with due allowance for the prevalence of the disease and the accuracy of the test. In the case of hypertension, most of these factors weigh in favor of screening and a low, close-to-normal dividing line for initial diagnosis. Prevalence is high, the test itself is harmless and inexpensive, and further testing and treatment are relatively harmless to someone who is incorrectly misclassified as hypertensive. Against this, and in favor of stricter diagnostic criteria although not necessarily less testing, the most likely mistake is that people who are misclassified will be diagnosed as mild hypertensives. Since the risk associated with blood pressures at this level is low, the possible gain from treatment for true positives is correspondingly low and may not outweigh the costs and risks of treating false positives. One analysis suggests that diagnostic criteria should be made stricter for the second and subsequent examination, precisely to reduce the chance that people with normal pressures will be treated for hypertension.[63]

Summarizing Costs and Benefits

The detection and treatment of hypertension are considerably more complicated to evaluate than are vaccines like those for smallpox or measles. There are more steps to take into account and commensurately more points at which the available information is incomplete. This discussion proceeds in stages, first considering some background on the measurement of costs and health effects, and then presenting estimates of the cost-effectiveness of hypertension treatment from a classic study by Weinstein and Stason.[64]

Costs

Each of the many steps required to detect and treat hypertension involves some cost. The population at risk must first be screened. Then those with elevated pressures must be examined a second and third time to confirm that their pressures are consistently high. If hypertension is confirmed at the third visit, the patient is examined and given lab tests to evaluate his or her general health and the extent of any hypertensive complications. The doctor may advise weight control and less salt, or if the patient's pressures are high enough or hypertensive complications

63. Rosner and Polk, "Implications of Blood Pressure Variability."
64. Weinstein and Stason, *Hypertension: A Policy Perspective.*

are present, drug treatment may start at once. At first, the patient will have to return frequently so that the doctor can monitor the decline in pressure and any drug reactions. Once the pressures have been reduced and a comfortable drug regimen established, visits may decline to as few as two or three a year.[65]

The cost per person for each step is rather small. Weinstein and Stason estimate that, in 1975, the first screening cost $6 per person. The second exam, assumed to take place at a doctor's office, cost $15. The third, including the physical exam and lab tests, cost about $100.[66] Treatment then averaged about $200 annually for drugs, extra physician visits, and lab tests; patients were assumed to average three more visits each year than if they had not been on medication. Treatment costs varied widely around the average, from about $160 to more than $400, depending primarily on the drug regimen. Treatment of side effects involves additional expense in some cases. Over the long term, of course, some of these costs will be balanced by savings from fewer strokes and heart attacks.

People who compare such low costs per person for a preventive measure with the high costs typical for acute care often conclude that prevention must be cost-effective, indeed, that it must save money. But costs are incurred at each step of detection and treatment, while benefits, including any savings, come only from long-term treatment of people correctly identified as hypertensive. The accumulation of costs as people are tested and treated means that programs that are inexpensive in terms of cost per person at each stage can be quite expensive per unit of ultimate benefit.

Among the major factors that influence costs are the prevalence of the condition, the diagnostic cutoff point, the accuracy of the screening test (and of the precursor condition as a predictor of serious illness), and people's willingness to undergo treatment.

—The less prevalent the condition in the population to be screened, the more it costs to find the people who have it. *Prevalence,* or the proportion of the population with the condition, is the relevant statistic for an initial screening. After that, *incidence*—the proportion of the population that has developed the condition since the last screening—is the appropriate statistic. Unless the time between screenings is very

65. Hypertension Study Group, "Guidelines for Detection," pp. 1086A–87A; and "Guidelines for the Treatment of Mild Hypertension."

66. Weinstein and Stason, *Hypertension: A Policy Perspective*, pp. 39, 82, 152–53.

long, the incidence of a slowly developing chronic disease like hypertension will be lower than its prevalence, and the yield of new cases from second and later screenings will be less than the yield from an initial screening.[67] The data given earlier on the distribution of blood pressures show the prevalence of high blood pressures.

—Choosing a higher cutoff point for screening (for example, 100 mm Hg rather than 90) raises the cost of finding hypertensives by reducing the prevalence of the condition being sought; but it lowers the costs at later stages, since fewer people progress to those stages and the ones who do derive greater benefit from treatment.

—As discussed earlier in the chapter, a third to a half of the people with high pressures at the first exam are likely to have pressures in the normal range at the second or third exam. These false positives involve costs for screening and rescreening but do not contribute to benefits. Most of them are sorted out before the treatment stage, but some are not.

—Some people diagnosed as hypertensive will not begin treatment or will discontinue it, contributing further to costs but not to benefits. Some will even continue to visit the doctor and buy medication, but will not take it.

Finally, how much is gained in return for this expense depends on the consequences of untreated disease and the efficacy of treatment. A highly effective treatment of a serious disease will produce large benefits to balance against the costs. A less successful treatment, or a successful treatment for a disease with only mild consequences, will yield less impressive benefits.

Health Effects

The analysts who evaluated measles vaccine made no attempt to produce a composite measure of all the health effects. They simply listed most of the major ones—numbers of lives saved, cases of retardation avoided, and so on. As other analysts have done, they could also have estimated the additional years of life represented by the saved lives. Where one outcome, such as lifesaving, is clearly the dominant one, the results of an evaluation can usefully be stated in terms of the cost per life saved, or per year of life.

67. Eddy, *Screening for Cancer,* chap. 3.

This simple approach begins to break down when several different health effects are important—particularly when the effects of alternatives are not directly comparable. Hypertension is a case in point. If hypertension is not treated, many people's lives will be shorter. Thus the obvious gain from treatment is the added years of life. But hypertension produces no symptoms for many years, while treatment often causes unpleasant side effects, so the patient who takes antihypertensive drugs may live longer but not feel as well as without treatment. Simply counting the years of life added by treatment overstates its benefits. Similarly, the simple approach gives no credit to treatments that improve people's health without extending their lives.

Somehow individuals balance the dissimilar effects of such alternatives in their own minds and arrive at a decision. Some reject treatment for their hypertension because of the side effects. Others, often with the concurrence of their doctors, decide not to pursue treatment aggressively, and stop short of reducing their blood pressures to the normal range. Still others value the potential health gains so highly that they are undeterred by side effects.

Analysts have recognized for some time that cost-effectiveness studies would be more useful if they could mimic this balancing process and produce a single, overall index of health effects that could be compared with costs. Considerable work has been done on the problem over the last ten or fifteen years.[68] The two requirements for such an index are an acceptable common unit for measuring health effects and some way of translating different health effects into the common unit.

The index used most often is the *quality-adjusted life-year,* recently renamed the *year of healthy life.* This approach makes a year of life in good health the standard unit and assigns it the value 1.0. The value is

68. Robert L. Berg, ed., *Health Status Indexes* (Chicago: Hospital Research and Educational Trust, 1973); George W. Torrance, "Social Preferences for Health States: An Empirical Evaluation of Three Measurement Techniques," *Socio-Economic Planning Sciences,* vol. 10 (1976), pp. 129–36; David L. Sackett and George W. Torrance, "The Utility of Different Health States as Perceived by the General Public," *Journal of Chronic Diseases,* vol. 31, no. 11 (1978), pp. 697–704; Stephen G. Pauker and Barbara J. McNeil, "Impact of Patient Preferences on the Selection of Therapy," *Journal of Chronic Diseases,* vol. 34, no. 2/3 (1981), pp. 77–86; George W. Torrance, Warren H. Thomas, and David L. Sackett, "A Utility Maximization Model for Evaluation of Health Care Programs," *Health Services Research,* vol. 7 (Summer 1972), pp. 118–33; and Joseph S. Pliskin, Donald S. Shepard, and Milton C. Weinstein, "Utility Functions for Life Years and Health Status," *Operations Research,* vol. 28 (January–February 1980), pp. 206–24.

assumed to be the same no matter who gains the year of healthy life. Whether a program adds ten healthy years to the life of a 30-year-old man, five healthy years to the lives of each of two people over 65, or one healthy year to the lives of each of ten people of different ages, the result is counted as a gain of ten healthy years. A year of life with some illness or disability is valued at a fraction of a healthy year and assigned a number between zero and 1.0. Death is usually assumed to be the worst possible state and given the value zero, although some people argue that extreme disability may be worse.

Weinstein and Stason used the concept of the year of healthy life in their study of hypertension. In principle, the value of a year on anti-hypertensive drugs should be derived by asking a sample of people how they would feel about it.[69] In practice, lacking a survey, Weinstein and Stason decided arbitrarily that most people would value a year of life with side effects from hypertensive medication as worth just under .99 of a year of healthy life. Thus an average person would be willing to give up only about 1 percent of his or her remaining life span, or about four days a year, to be free of side effects; if the person's remaining life span with treatment is expected to be twenty years, this represents a reduction of two and a half months.

The idea of the year of healthy life is straightforward enough, but as yet neither the concept nor the methods proposed for its application have been completely worked out or accepted. Analysts have used surveys to try to discover the values people place on different states of health. Several methods are available to present people with choices that will elicit these values. Perhaps the most clear-cut is the "time trade-off" method, in which respondents are asked to imagine that they can expect to live a specified number of years in a specified state of health, and to say how many years of life they would be willing to trade for excellent health during the remaining years. For example, if a respondent valued seven years of excellent health as highly as ten years on dialysis, the implicit value of a year on dialysis would be .70 of a healthy year. Such questions must be carefully phrased—the state of health to be considered must be described fully so that each respondent pictures the situation the same way and does not fill in a sketchy description with different details.[70]

69. Weinstein and Stason, *Hypertension: A Policy Perspective* p. 26.
70. Several analysts have examined the assumptions about decisionmaking implicit

Since the completion of Weinstein and Stason's study, further advances have been made in the measurement of preferences for states of health. Several groups of researchers, working independently, have made the concept of the healthy year easier to apply by defining health, not in terms of specific diseases, but in terms of ability to function. In one variation on this approach, Bush, Kaplan, and their colleagues distinguish a number of aspects of function and accompanying symptom or problem complexes.[71] For example, an individual might be confined to bed (the level of function) and suffering from coughing, wheezing, or shortness of breath (the symptom/problem complex). The researchers asked a large sample of people in San Diego, California, to place values on various combinations of function levels and symptoms; the results differed very little among social and economic groups and, of particular importance, were virtually the same for low-income and high-income respondents.[72]

Specific diseases can be described in terms of the levels of function and symptoms, and the length of time each of those levels of function and symptoms lasts. For example, if the person confined to bed with shortness of breath has a cold, the impairment will last only a few days; if he or she has chronic bronchitis, much more time will be affected. By defining different conditions in terms of a common set of elements this approach helps to maintain and test the consistency of valuations of diverse states of health. Further, the same survey results can be used for analyses of very different diseases by using the values for the states of health associated with those diseases; new surveys need not be done each time.

Kaplan and his colleagues have carried out further tests of the validity of the year of healthy life and of their methods of obtaining values. In a study of patients being treated for chronic obstructive lung disease, they found that the patients' valuations of their state of health correlated well

---

in the concept to determine whether they are consistent with those of utility theory—the economic theory of how people make decisions—and with the empirical evidence. In general, the concept is, or can be made to be, consistent with utility theory. See, for example, Torrance, "Social Preferences for Health States."

71. Robert M. Kaplan, "Quality of Life Measurement," in Paul Karoly, ed., *Measurement Strategies in Health Psychology* (Wiley, 1985), pp. 115–46.

72. Robert M. Kaplan, J. W. Bush, and Charles C. Berry, "The Reliability, Stability, and Generalizability of a Health Status Index," in American Statistical Association, *Proceedings of the American Statistical Association Social Statistics Section* (Washington, D.C.: ASA, 1978), pp. 704–09.

with medical tests of their lung function, and correlated best with the medical measure considered to be the best, the forced expiratory volume in one second.[73] In another study they tested the assumption, implicit in their approach, that the distinct characteristics of health are additive, that is, that a particular symptom or function will make the same difference in the overall valuation of health regardless of the other symptoms or functions with which it is combined (for example, a fever will always reduce the value of a given health status by .07). Analysis of individuals' ratings of various states of health supported the additivity assumption.[74]

Researchers at the University of Washington in Seattle have pursued the same approach—defining health in terms of the ability to function rather than in terms of disease—with a somewhat different twist.[75] Using people's descriptions of the effects illness had on them, they developed questions that explore psychosocial as well as physical function. For example, their questionnaire, modified and refined in the course of many trials, asks not only about the person's ability to walk, work, and undertake other common activities, but about his or her emotional state, mental alertness, and willingness to participate in social activities. This Sickness Impact Profile, as it is called, has been tested repeatedly for consistency, stability, and agreement with other measures of health. It too assigns numerical values to each aspect of health so that an overall index of improvement or deterioration can be calculated. In several clinical studies it has shown that it can reveal important differences in health under various therapeutic regimens.

The concept of the year of healthy life is an important contribution to the evaluation of health programs. The usefulness of cost-effectiveness analysis increases as it permits comparison of a wider and wider range of alternatives—for example, not just several policies toward hypertension, but measles vaccination versus treatment of hypertension versus policies toward still other health problems. A common unit for measuring health effects is essential for such comparisons.

73. Robert M. Kaplan, Catherine J. Atkins, and Richard Timms, "Validity of a Quality of Well-Being Scale as an Outcome Measure in Chronic Obstructive Pulmonary Disease," *Journal of Chronic Diseases*, vol. 37, no. 2 (1984), pp. 85–95.

74. Robert M. Kaplan, "Human Preference Measurement for Health Decisions and the Evaluation of Long-Term Care," in Robert L. Kane and Rosalie A. Kane, eds., *Values and Long-Term Care* (Lexington Books, 1982), pp. 157–88.

75. Marilyn Bergner and others, "The Sickness Impact Profile: Development and Final Revision of a Health Status Measure," *Medical Care*, vol. 19 (August 1981), pp. 787–805.

The Cost-Effectiveness of Treating Hypertension

The cost per year of healthy life gained by finding and treating hypertension can vary dramatically with the characteristics of the patient, the choices made about treatment, and the assumptions about areas of uncertainty. Although a single estimate for the most common set of conditions is useful, it is still more useful to estimate costs under a series of different sets of conditions in order to show which are most (or least) costly and which areas of uncertainty are most important to the results. This approach helps guide not only investment in medical care, but investment in research to address some of the uncertainties.

Weinstein and Stason followed this plan in their study of hypertension.[76] They made the comparison of different conditions vastly easier by summarizing their calculations of costs and effects more succinctly than was done in the study of measles vaccination discussed in chapter 2, which considered only one set of assumptions. For each set of conditions, all costs were added together, and so were all health effects (after they had been translated into years of healthy life). The costs were then divided by the gain in healthy years of life so that the result could be presented in terms of a single number—the cost per year of healthy life. This number is the cost-effectiveness ratio. Formally stated:

$$\text{cost-effectiveness ratio} = \frac{\text{total costs}}{\text{total years of healthy life gained}}$$

$$= \text{cost per healthy year}$$

Because the cost-effectiveness of screening depends on the cost-effectiveness of the ensuing treatment, Weinstein and Stason first focused on treatment alone. They calculated the additional costs and the health effects of drug therapy and compared them with leaving hypertension untreated and treating the resulting disease.

Specifically, the total costs of treating hypertension were estimated as the sum of

—the cost of the treatment itself, including drugs, visits to doctors, and lab tests;

—plus the cost of treating the side effects of the drugs;

—minus the saving in medical costs because disease is prevented;

—plus the cost of medical care in the years of life added by treatment.

All costs were measured in 1975 dollars. They were limited to medical

76. Weinstein and Stason, *Hypertension: A Policy Perspective.*

care because no other costs—such as those of institutionalization, included in the study of measles vaccine—were known to be important.

As discussed in chapter 2, it is appropriate to include ordinary medical expenses in added years of life only when the main concern of the study is the effect on the medical sector, and thus on total expenditures for medical care. If the study adopts the broader perspective of society in general, only medical expenses for hypertension treatment (and any savings that flow directly from it) are relevant. Medical costs in added years of life are a major item in some studies. Fortunately, in Weinstein and Stason's estimates they rarely account for even as much as 10 percent of the total cost per year of healthy life, so the results can be interpreted as approximately correct from the social perspective.[77]

Total health effects were estimated as the sum of the following elements, each translated into years of healthy life:

—the added years of life expected from treatment;

—plus improvements in health during years that would have been lived anyway, because nonfatal disease is also prevented by treatment;

—minus any deterioration in health because of the side effects of treatment.

As discussed above, side effects were valued at four days a year, that is, four days were subtracted from the health gains for every year of treatment. Values were assigned to improvements in health on the basis of experts' estimates of the extent of disability that would be caused by stroke and myocardial infarction (heart attack) and the authors' own guesses about how people would value life with disability compared with good health.[78]

The estimates of health effects required a considerable amount of work. First the authors estimated the relation between diastolic blood pressure and mortality using data from the Framingham study. They then developed alternative assumptions about the effect of treatment on this mortality. The extreme possibility, of course, is that treatment reduces the mortality rate of hypertensives to the same level observed in people whose blood pressures are naturally low, but this has not been proved.[79] For most of their estimates, Weinstein and Stason used the

77. Ibid., pp. 75–76.

78. Ibid., pp. 34, 69.

79. Lew in "The New Build and Blood Pressure Study" reports that a small study of treated male hypertensives included as part of the larger study found that those whose pressures were reduced below 150/100 had a death rate about the same as men with normal pressures.

intermediate assumption that the benefit of treatment is greater for young people than for older ones, and greater the longer treatment is continued, but that a treated hypertensive can never achieve quite the same good health as someone whose blood pressure is naturally low. They called this the age-varying partial benefit assumption. The authors also assumed for most of their estimates that patients take their medication faithfully and achieve the maximum possible benefit.[80]

Both the costs and effects of treating hypertension occur over many years. It is usually assumed that present health effects, like present dollars, are valued more highly than future ones. To represent this valuation, Weinstein and Stason discounted costs and effects at 5 percent a year. Thus the cost-effectiveness ratio gives the discounted lifetime cost per discounted year of healthy life gained. The choice of a discount rate, discussed more fully in chapter 5, is important because discounting often reduces health benefits, most of which occur years after treatment begins, more than it reduces costs. The higher the rate of discount, the higher the discounted lifetime cost per year of healthy life.

Estimates from Weinstein and Stason's study show that the cost-effectiveness of treating hypertension varies considerably depending on the sex of the patient and the age when treatment begins, even when all other factors, such as the yearly cost of drugs, are constant (table 3-3). For individuals whose diastolic pressure is reduced from 110 to 90, the estimates range from a low of $3,270 per year of healthy life for 20-year-old men, to $16,330 for men aged 60 (recall that the estimates are in 1975 dollars). By contrast, the cost for women falls with age, because hypertension seems to cause less damage in women, especially when they are young. There are also substantial differences in cost associated with differences in the level of blood pressure before and during treatment: this is indicated by the addendum shown for men and women aged 50. In general, the lower the pressure at the outset, the higher the cost of producing a healthy year of life through treatment.

Table 3-4 demonstrates the effects of varying some of the study's more important assumptions one at a time. The reference case, which is the point of comparison, includes the assumptions that the efficacy of treatment varies with age and length of treatment (age-varying partial benefit), that treatment costs $200 per year, that a year with side effects is about .01 less valuable than a healthy year, and that patients are in

80. Similar procedures were used to estimate declines in morbidity, that is, improvements in health, as a result of treatment.

Table 3-3. Cost-Effectiveness of Reducing Diastolic Pressure from 110 to 90 with Medication, by Sex and Age[a]

1975 dollars

	Cost per year of healthy life	
Age[b]	Men	Women
20	3,270	8,490
30	4,000	6,520
40	5,190	5,990
50	6,870	6,000
60	16,330	5,030

Addendum: Cost-effectiveness of medication for 50-year-olds, by pressure
Reduction

	Men	Women
90 to 80	33,880	18,640
100 to 85	12,820	9,290
110 to 90	6,870	6,000
120 to 95	3,920	3,840

Source: Milton C. Weinstein and William B. Stason, *Hypertension: A Policy Perspective* (Harvard University Press, 1976), pp. 75 and 76.

a. Assumptions common to all estimates: age-varying partial benefit; treatment costs $200 a year; side effects valued at .01 of a healthy year (four days a year); complete compliance with treatment regimen; discount rate of 5 percent a year.

b. Age at the beginning of treatment.

complete compliance with their prescribed treatment regimens. The estimates shown are for 50-year-olds (men and women) with diastolic pressures before treatment of 110, which are reduced to 90 by treatment.

One point evident from the table is that costs can vary two- and threefold when even a single condition is changed to another plausible value. For example, if treatment is fully effective—that is, if people whose pressure is reduced to a particular level by drugs experience mortality rates no higher than those of people whose pressure is naturally at the same level—the cost per healthy year is much less than under the age-varying partial benefit assumption. For men, it drops from $6,900 to $2,300; for women, from $6,000 to $3,000. The cost per healthy year is also substantially lower if the outlay for treating hypertension is $100 a year rather than $200—and substantially higher if treatment costs $300 a year. Changing other variables produces similarly large effects.

If side effects trouble people more than Weinstein and Stason assume in their reference case—if people would be willing to give up .02, or eight days, of each year rather than .01—the health gains from treatment are substantially less, and the cost per healthy year correspondingly greater. How completely people adhere to the treatment regimen is also important. If patients do not take all the prescribed medication, and thus do

Table 3-4. Cost-Effectiveness of Treating Hypertension with Medication in 50-Year-Olds, under Alternative Assumptions[a]
1975 dollars

Assumption	Cost per year of healthy life	
	Men	Women
Reference case[b]	6,900	6,000
Change:		
Treatment confers full benefit	2,300	3,000
Treatment costs		
$100 a year	3,300	2,600
$300 a year	10,200	9,300
Side effects valued at .02	10,500	9,000
Incomplete compliance with treatment regimen		
Minimum cost[c]	9,300	8,000
Maximum cost[d]	14,900	13,200

Source: Weinstein and Stason, *Hypertension: A Policy Perspective*, figs. 2.6, 2.7, 2.17, 2.18, and tables 4.2 and 4.3.

a. Age at the beginning of treatment. All cases assume that treatment reduces diastolic pressure from 110 to 90.

b. Assumes age-varying partial benefit; treatment costs $200 a year; side effects valued at .01 of a healthy year (four days a year); complete compliance with treatment regimen; discount rate of 5 percent a year.

c. Patient continues to visit doctor but does not take the full amount of medication prescribed and reduces purchases accordingly.

d. Patient continues to visit doctor and buys all the medication prescribed but does not take it all.

not achieve the full benefit of treatment, costs are incurred without the hoped-for gain and the cost per healthy year is higher. The estimates assume that these patients continue to visit the doctor at the same rate as other patients; the lower estimate assumes that they buy only as much medicine as they take, while the higher one assumes they buy the full amount prescribed by the doctor, thus wasting the part they do not take.

The estimates in tables 3-3 and 3-4 are solely for treatment. In effect, they include only those costs that would be incurred if physicians treated hypertensives who came to their attention in the course of visits for other reasons. But since the early 1970s, numerous community programs have been created to screen for hypertension, programs that actively search for people who are unaware of their hypertension. By their nature, these programs are not aimed at narrow age-groups, so Weinstein and Stason estimated the costs of screening all adults; thus the estimates cannot be compared directly with the more detailed estimates for treatment. They estimate the cost of screening *and* treating all adults with moderate or severe hypertension at $7,000 per healthy year, compared with $4,850 for treatment alone. If the program aims to find people with mild hypertension as well, specifically everyone with a diastolic pressure of 95 or higher, screening plus treatment costs $8,600 per year (there is no comparable estimate for treatment alone). If patients do not take all the prescribed medicine, the cost per healthy year is substantially higher for either kind of program.[81]

The tables indicate that a large number of factors are important to the cost-effectiveness of treating hypertension. In real-life situations, where several conditions, not just one, may vary from the reference conditions, the cost per year of healthy life could be much higher or much lower than any of the numbers shown in the tables. One conclusion, however, is consistently supported by the estimates—screening for and treating hypertension adds to medical expenditures. Given that, whether treatment is considered worthwhile must depend on the particular situation, which determines the cost per healthy year, and on the value placed on an additional year of healthy life.

Some Further Issues

Unlike vaccination, screening by itself has no health benefit—it simply identifies people who can benefit from treatment. Thus to evaluate screening one must evaluate the entire sequence of events from screening through treatment, and the benefits, risks, and costs at each step in the sequence. Eddy has observed that "the number of important factors that must be considered simply exceeds the capacity of the unaided mind" and that "a few oversimplifications or mistakes can cost millions of lives and billions of dollars."[82]

Health effects and costs can vary dramatically for different screening tests, or even for the same test under different conditions. Although the analysis of hypertension presented in this chapter illustrates many of the important factors, it by no means illustrates all of them. This final section touches on some of the issues omitted or slighted in the case of hypertension. As in chapter 2, it helps to organize the discussion in terms of populations and frequency, risk, uncertainty, individual values, and time.

81. These figures illustrate dramatically that an inexpensive test applied to a large number of people, most of whom do not have the disease, can generate large costs per unit of ultimate health effect. However, in its 1984 report, the Joint National Committee on Detection, Evaluation, and Treatment of High Blood Pressure stated that, since most adults now have their pressures measured in the course of routine visits to doctors, "mass screening programs for this purpose are seldom indicated." "1984 Report," p. 1045.

82. David M. Eddy, "The Economics of Cancer Prevention and Detection: Getting More for Less," Cancer, vol. 47 (March 1, 1981), pp. 1200, 1201.

The costs and effects of a preventive measure depend in large part on the size of the *population* involved in the program and on the *frequency* with which the measure must be applied to that population. In vaccination programs, frequency is usually far less important than population size, since a single vaccination lasts many years, even a lifetime. But screening usually aims at detecting a condition that can develop at any time—the person who does not have it today may develop it tomorrow. To be certain of detecting the condition as early as possible, it would be necessary to test for it often, perhaps every month or even every day. The critical determinant of the best frequency for a screening test turns out to be the length of time the condition exists in a detectable, preclinical state.[83] If this preclinical period is short, frequent tests will be necessary to catch the condition early. If it is long, fewer tests will be sufficient.

As complicated as the analysis by Weinstein and Stason is, it does not address the issue of the frequency of testing for hypertension. Instead, it evaluates the case in which the adult population is screened for the first time and those found to have hypertension are treated, leaving aside the difficult question of the costs and effects of different schedules for retesting adults found to be normal in the initial screening.

Eddy has analyzed exactly this question of frequency for a variety of cancer screening tests.[84] For example, using the best clinical information on the natural history, detection, and treatment of cervical cancer, he found that administering Pap tests to adult women every three or four years would produce almost as much health benefit, measured in years of life saved, as administering them every year, and at less than a third the cost.[85] The preclinical course of cervical cancer is so long that, even with tests only every three or four years, it can be detected long before it would become clinically apparent.

Until this analysis, the American Cancer Society had advocated annual Pap tests. But in 1980, it recommended that young adult women should be given two tests, a year apart, and if both were normal, subsequent tests should be given every three years.[86] At the same time,

---

83. Ibid., pp. 1202–04.
84. See Eddy, *Screening for Cancer*, pp. 244–45; Eddy, "The Economics of Cancer Prevention and Detection"; and David M. Eddy, "Appropriateness of Cervical Cancer Screening," *Gynecologic Oncology*, vol. 12 (October 1981), pp. S168–87.
85. Eddy, "The Economics of Cancer Prevention and Detection."
86. American Cancer Society, *Guidelines for the Cancer-related Health Checkup: Recommendations and Rationale* (New York: ACS, 1980), p. 5. Note that Eddy's analysis does not show that annual Pap tests bring no additional health benefit, only that the benefit is very small and costly. From the point of view of the whole population,

based on related analyses, it recommended changes in the frequencies of other cancer screening tests and the elimination of chest x-rays for lung cancer.

The issues of population and *risk* become intertwined when, in an effort to achieve the best balance of benefits, risks, and costs, advisory groups try to identify high-risk groups for screening. But Eddy notes that so-called high-risk groups often do not face risks very much higher than the rest of the population; and even when their risks are much higher, they may represent a small part of the total population and of the total amount of disease. To limit screening to them would miss most of the disease and thus most of the benefit of early detection. Adjusting frequency can be the answer—if everyone is tested, but less often, most of the health benefit is retained, and costs are kept at a reasonable level.

The evaluation of a screening test must consider not only the risks of the disease, but those of the test itself, and of subsequent tests and treatment. An important risk is that patients will be misclassified and either fail to receive treatment when they have the disease, or undergo further testing, and possibly even treatment, when they do not. Screening for colon cancer is a case in which the risk of misclassification, specifically the risk of false-positive test results, dominates the evaluation.[87] The initial screening test—the stool occult blood test—is very cheap. But even under the best of conditions, about 1.5 percent of people who do not have cancer will produce (false) positive test results.[88] The expense of the additional tests required to check the initial diagnosis—about $700 in 1981 for sigmoidoscopy, barium enema, colonoscopy, and x-ray studies of the upper gastrointestinal tract—turns out to be by far the largest item in the total cost of a screening program.

The information about risks, effects, and costs needed to evaluate a screening test is inevitably measured with *uncertainty*. The estimates in

---

the same money could buy much more health if it were applied elsewhere—for example, to screening women who have never been screened. But an individual concerned about her own health might prefer to continue having annual tests. It is partly for this reason that several medical groups continue to recommend annual tests. In a recent consensus development conference, the National Institutes of Health refused to choose between annual tests and tests every three years. National Institutes of Health, *Consensus Development Conference Summaries*, vol. 3 (Bethesda, Md.: NIH, 1980), p. 27.

87. Eddy, "The Economics of Cancer Prevention and Detection," p. 1206.

88. And if the stool test is given without instructing the patient on the proper diet to be followed during the test period, the false-positive rate, and thus the costs and needless risks, can be much higher.

tables 3-3 and 3-4 of the cost of hypertension treatment under different circumstances indicate how important this uncertainty can be. Should even a single value used in the reference case be off, the cost can double, or halve. As noted in the case of vaccinations, this uncertainty is more important when the gain from a screening program is estimated to be small; better information might show it to yield no gain at all. Also as in the case of vaccinations, some pieces of information—such as the long-term results of antihypertensive drug therapy—are impossible to measure precisely, or at all, before the program is applied to the whole population.

With more steps than vaccination, screening programs involve more points at which *individual values* can influence people's decisions. One of these points is the decision to take the screening test in the first place. Eddy reports that people often feel strongly about the physical and psychological discomfort, the inconvenience, and the time involved in being screened;[89] sometimes these factors deter them from being tested. Nor can this phenomenon be dismissed as due to the ignorance of patients who fail to value the potential gains properly: medical specialists also give heavy weight to the negative aspects of screening tests.

Finally, *time* affects decisions about screening, especially when its benefits follow many years after the costs. Screening of children aimed at improving health in adulthood offers an extreme example. In one study analysts found that time, represented by the discount rate, dominated their evaluation of screening for high cholesterol levels in children. They noted that "when intervention can be delayed—that is, undertaken at a time closer to the time at which benefits are realized—with little or no decrease in benefits, discounting will lead us to take advantage of that delay instead of shouldering intervention costs at an unnecessarily early time."[90]

89. Eddy, "The Economics of Cancer Prevention and Detection," pp. 1206–07.
90. Donald M. Berwick, Shan Cretin, and Emmett B. Keeler, *Cholesterol, Children, and Heart Disease: An Analysis of Alternatives* (Oxford University Press, 1980), p. 277.

chapter four **Lifestyle**

The choices individuals make about their personal habits—what to eat, whether to smoke, how much to exercise, when to sleep—can affect their health and longevity. These choices have attracted the interest of medical researchers and policymakers in recent years. Many of them believe that "lifestyle" is the most promising area for preventive efforts.

A growing body of research supports the link between lifestyle and health and attempts to pin down more precisely what is involved. In a study unique in its size and scope, researchers at the University of California demonstrated the truth of the general proposition: lifestyles that fit the accepted notions of healthy living are indeed associated with better health and lower death rates. The study began in 1965 with a survey of adults then living in Alameda County, California. Almost 7,000 people answered a questionnaire about their health and personal habits. The healthiest people usually followed most or all of seven common-sense practices: they slept seven to eight hours a night, ate breakfast and rarely snacked between meals, maintained a reasonable weight, did not smoke, drank alcohol in moderation if at all, and often took part in some sort of physical activity.[1] Each practice taken alone contributed to better health and the combined effect of all of them was substantial. In a 1972 article based on the study, the authors concluded that the health of people who followed all seven good health practices "was consistently about the same as [that of people] 30 years younger who followed few or none of these practices."[2]

The researchers kept track of deaths in the survey group for a number

1. Even people who took weekend auto trips, not a strenuous form of exercise, had better-than-average health, but those who participated in hunting or fishing did not.
2. Nedra B. Belloc and Lester Breslow, "Relationship of Physical Health Status and Health Practices," *Preventive Medicine*, vol. 1, no. 3 (1972), p. 419.

of years. Between 1965 and 1974 the death rate among men who followed all seven good health practices was only 28 percent that of men who followed three or fewer.[3] For women, the comparable statistic was 43 percent. Further examination showed that people with numerous social ties had lower death rates than those with fewer, even when they followed the same health practices; marriage and contacts with close friends and relatives were most important, but church and group memberships also contributed to this result.[4] The final report on the project confirmed the earlier results, with the exception that breakfast and snacking between meals did not turn out to be important when the other health practices, and social ties, were taken into account.[5]

This research provides a backdrop for studies that focus on a single aspect of lifestyle. Such studies try to pin down why a particular practice is helpful or harmful, and precisely what its effects are under different conditions. Bit by bit, they are producing the information necessary to evaluate individual health practices and to make better personal and public choices.

Over the past several decades, for example, a great deal has been learned about the effects of smoking—which diseases it causes and how long they take to develop, the differences between heavy and light smokers, the specific constituents of tobacco that cause the damage, and how long it takes for the effects to wear off once a smoker gives up the habit. Recent research has begun to explore the effects of smoking on nonsmokers, particularly the children, spouses, and co-workers of smokers. The questions that can be asked about diet are even more complex. Research on the subject is accumulating rapidly, with particular interest in the links between components of diet and cancer.

With the burgeoning interest in and evidence about the health effects of lifestyle, a logical next step is to evaluate the cost-effectiveness of changing lifestyles. Claims have been made that changes in lifestyle are among the most cost-effective of ways to improve health and, further, that more emphasis on them will reduce medical expenditures. But in

3. Lester Breslow and James E. Enstrom, "Persistence of Health Habits and Their Relationship to Mortality," *Preventive Medicine*, vol. 9, no. 4 (1980), pp. 478–79. Death rates were adjusted for differences in age between the groups.
4. Lisa F. Berkman and S. Leonard Syme, "Social Networks, Host Resistance, and Mortality: A Nine-Year Follow-up Study of Alameda County Residents," *American Journal of Epidemiology*, vol. 109 (February 1979), pp. 186–204.
5. Lisa F. Berkman and Lester Breslow, *Health and Ways of Living: The Alameda County Study* (Oxford University Press, 1983), pp. 89–90, 214–18.

fact there are very few analyses of changes in lifestyle, and fewer still that meet the standards attained by the best studies of immunization and screening. One reason is that a good cost-effectiveness analysis requires good scientific evidence about effects. The evidence about subjects like diet and exercise is just reaching the point where it can support such studies.

This chapter describes how to set about a cost-effectiveness analysis of a change in lifestyle, using exercise as an example. The first step is to gather the evidence about the health effects and costs of exercise. This information must then be combined in ways that show its cost-effectiveness under different circumstances. One of the obvious distinctions between changes in lifestyle and vaccination, or screening, is that many of the decisions, and many of the costs, occur outside the medical sector. As a result, the methods developed for analyses of medical services must be modified somewhat. These new issues are discussed.

Two aspects of any preventive measure can be evaluated—the cost-effectiveness of the measure itself as a way to improve health, and the cost-effectiveness of ways to persuade people to adopt the measure. Both are legitimate issues for analysis and legitimate concerns of public policy. But the cost-effectiveness of the measure as a way to improve health comes first logically because efforts to persuade depend on and include it. In an analogous situation, that of screening for hypertension, Weinstein and Stason had to evaluate the cost-effectiveness of treatment before they could evaluate alternative screening programs.

The discussion here focuses primarily on the cost-effectiveness of exercise as a way to improve health. No evaluation of this fundamental issue has been done. Until one is, it is impossible to know whether exercise is truly as good an investment in health as it appears to be to its supporters, or how it compares with other preventive measures that might be the object of public policy. If exercise is found to be a good investment in health, the next question is the appropriate and cost-effective role of public (or private) institutions in promoting it. The chapter refers to this second set of questions from time to time but does not go into detail about it.

Health Effects of Exercise—The Evidence

For many years doctors and researchers thought that vigorous exercise was bad for adults. The prevailing view was that human beings were subject to wear and tear, much like machines; the harder they worked themselves the sooner they would wear out.[6] A British study published in 1953 challenged this view.[7] The authors compared London bus drivers with bus conductors, who got considerable exercise climbing the stairs of the double-decker buses to collect tickets. Even after correction for differences in age, the conductors were found to have heart disease only 70 percent as often as the drivers, and heart attacks only half as often.

The effect of exercise on heart disease has continued to be the major focus of research, and a great many studies have been carried out since this paper was published. The earliest ones suffered from a number of serious defects.[8] They usually failed to correct for other factors related to heart disease; people who get less exercise are also more likely to smoke, be overweight, and have high blood pressure and high cholesterol.[9] Further, people with heart disease or characteristics conducive to it may choose to be inactive, so that lack of exercise is the consequence of the disease rather than its cause—this problem is referred to as self-selection. Finally, the early studies used very crude indicators of exercise. Accurately measuring the amount of exercise people get is difficult, much more so than measuring their blood pressures, for example. These studies often accepted job titles as an index of exercise, and examined only exercise on the job or only recreational exercise, assuming that the omitted area was not a source of important differences among individuals.

Studies published more recently have fewer problems. Although none have randomly assigned people to exercise or nonexercise—the best way to ensure that other factors do not muddy the results—they have been more careful to control for these other factors in the design of the study and in the subsequent analysis, and to measure exercise more precisely. To reduce the problems caused by self-selection, they have

6. John O. Holloszy, "Exercise, Health, and Aging: A Need for More Information," *Medicine and Science in Sports and Exercise*, vol. 15, no. 1 (1983), p. 1; and Roy J. Shephard, *Physical Activity and Aging* (London: Croom Helm, 1978), pp. 35–37.

7. For a discussion of the study, see Nancy A. Rigotti, Gregory S. Thomas, and Alexander Leaf, "Exercise and Coronary Heart Disease," *Annual Review of Medicine*, vol. 34 (1983), p. 394.

8. Ibid., pp. 394–95.

9. The study of bus drivers and conductors was criticized on these grounds. After reexamining the data, the authors discovered that, on average, conductors were thinner than drivers at the time they were hired, a difference that would give them an advantage even without the extra exercise. They adjusted the results for this difference and still found that conductors had less heart disease and fewer heart attacks. Ibid.

generally used a prospective design, identifying active and sedentary individuals who do not have heart disease at the outset of the study and following them over a period of years to observe the rates at which they develop heart disease. Of the large number of prospective studies now available, two are considered to provide the most reliable evidence—a study of San Francisco longshoremen and a study of Harvard alumni.

Benefits

The study of San Francisco longshoremen followed nearly 4,000 men for a period of twenty-two years.[10] The men were between 35 and 74 years of age when the study began in 1951. Union rules helped to minimize the problem of self-selection: all the men had to do heavy work for five years before they were eligible for other assignments. The researchers kept careful records of other factors known to be related to heart disease. Exercise during time off the job was not recorded, but the work on the job was so strenuous that it seems reasonable to assume that this omission is not important—the men got most of their exercise at work.

About 10 percent of the longshoremen died of heart attacks during the study. The men who used 8,500 calories[11] or more during a week of work had significantly fewer deaths from heart attack than those who were less active. Even when other factors were controlled for, the difference was substantial (the other factors were smoking, hypertension, high cholesterol, overweight, diabetes, prior heart disease, and job transfers). In this controlled analysis, the risk of death from heart attack declined steadily as the amount of physical activity increased: those who used 9,500 calories a week had half the risk of those who used only 4,750. A rather different calculation produced a similar result: the researchers estimated that if all the longshoremen had worked at a level of 8,500 calories or more, deaths from heart attack would have been cut in half. But it should be noted that all the longshoremen, even the ones counted as "less active," were exercising at levels beyond the requirements of

10. Gregory S. Thomas and others, *Exercise and Health: The Evidence and the Implications* (Cambridge, Mass.: Oelgeschlager, Gunn and Hain, 1981), pp. 30–34, 42–47; and Rigotti and others, "Exercise and Coronary Heart Disease," pp. 395–96.

11. The technical term, used in many discussions of the results, is *kilocalories*. This is the unit used to measure the energy value of foods and is known to the layman simply as *calories*.

most jobs. While the study shows that exercise is beneficial, it says little about the levels of exercise most adults get, or might aspire to.

The study of Harvard alumni focused on exercise during leisure time in a group of men most of whom had sedentary jobs or were retired.[12] Men who had entered Harvard between 1916 and 1950 were followed for six to ten years during the period 1962–72. The study counted all first heart attacks, whether fatal or not, and found that men who used 2,000 calories or more a week in their recreational exercise had significantly fewer attacks than those who used under 2,000.[13] The difference remained substantial even after correction for other factors related to heart disease.[14] And here too the risk of heart attack declined steadily as the amount of exercise increased, at least up to 4,000 calories a week— showing that some exercise is better than none, and more is better than less.[15] The study distinguished vigorous sports from less vigorous forms of exercise and found that, for a given expenditure of calories, vigorous sports reduced risk more.[16] At exactly 2,000 calories, for example, men who engaged in vigorous sports had about two-thirds the risk of those who did virtually nothing, while those who engaged in less vigorous activities had 75 to 80 percent of the risk.

Several points about these two studies deserve comment. Like most studies of the subject, they observed middle-aged men; much less is known about the effects of exercise on women and older people. They also illustrate a problem in identifying the true effect of exercise. No one knows exactly how exercise protects against heart disease; some research indicates that it may do so in part by helping to control cholesterol, blood pressure, and some of the other factors associated with heart disease. Thus analyses that correct for these factors understate the effect of exercise, since they give it credit only for that part produced through

12. Thomas and others, *Exercise and Health,* pp. 35–41, 48–54; and Rigotti and others, "Exercise and Coronary Heart Disease."

13. Thomas and his colleagues estimate that the men probably used an additional 4,500 to 5,000 calories in the course of their work. This is useful for comparisons with the study of longshoremen. They do not, however, suggest how much should be added to the longshoremen's totals to represent their leisure-time exercise.

14. The other factors were smoking, high blood pressure, a personal history of stroke or diabetes, a parent with a history of heart attack or high blood pressure, overweight, and short stature.

15. Thomas and others, *Exercise and Health,* p. 51.

16. Vigorous sports were defined as those requiring about ten calories a minute, such as running or swimming. Other, lighter activities were estimated to require about five calories a minute.

means as yet unidentified. Analyses that do not correct for these factors overstate the effect, since there are other determinants of cholesterol, high blood pressure, and so on.

Another serious limitation is that these studies, like most others, examine only heart disease, and not always the same measure of heart disease—some count heart attacks, some only deaths from heart attacks, and some use other measures. The point was made in chapter 3 that more comprehensive measures of health effect—all deaths, all sickness—are necessary for reliable judgments. The true effect of exercise is larger than these studies indicate if exercise also reduces death and illness from other causes. It is smaller if the beneficial impact on heart disease is offset by bad outcomes elsewhere. A Finnish study suggests that the first case may be true: deaths from all causes were fewer for those who exercised.[17] The study was, however, done in two Finnish counties where mortality from heart disease is exceptionally high, so alternative causes of death are much less important than in other parts of the world.

Even if exercise does little to reduce deaths from causes other than heart disease, it has a wide range of other potential benefits, benefits that have more to do with the quality of life than its duration. Some of them are substantiated by good, scientific evidence, while others are not much more than reasonable expectations. Many are succinctly summarized by the statement "regular exercise can increase endurance, strength, suppleness, and skill."[18]

Exercise increases physical working capacity and thus helps reduce fatigue; over periods of eight hours or more people can work at only 20 to 25 percent of their maximum capacity, and when that capacity is low, fatigue can become a chronic problem.[19] Exercise can reduce some of the difficulties associated with pregnancy, particularly fatigue and back pain.[20] More generally, by strengthening the supporting muscles, it can

17. Jukka T. Salonen, Pekka Puska, and Jaakko Tuomilehto, "Physical Activity and Risk of Myocardial Infarction, Cerebral Stroke and Death: A Longitudinal Study in Eastern Finland," *American Journal of Epidemiology*, vol. 115 (April 1982), pp. 526–37.

18. Archie Young, "Exercise in the Prevention of Disease and Disability," in Muir Gray and Godfrey Fowler, eds., *Preventive Medicine in General Practice* (Oxford University Press, 1983), p. 160.

19. William L. Haskell and Steven N. Blair, "The Physical Activity Component of Health Promotion in Occupational Settings," *Public Health Reports*, vol. 95 (March–April 1980), pp. 111–12.

20. P. Edwards and others, "Fitness and Pregnancy: A Round Table Discussion," *Canadian Journal of Public Health*, vol. 74 (March–April 1983), pp. 86–90.

prevent or relieve back and joint problems; the joint problems that accompany arthritis and old age are complicated by weak muscles.[21] Exercise helps counteract chronic lung disease by strengthening the respiratory muscles and raising the level at which breathlessness occurs.[22] It helps control maturity-onset diabetes[23] and reverse the bone loss that occurs particularly among older women.[24] Finally, it promotes weight control and may relieve anxiety and depression;[25] certainly, many people will attest that it makes them feel better.

Many of the conditions that may be improved by exercise—joint problems, lung disease, bone loss—are common among the elderly. Thus it is argued that exercise should be able to make a major contribution to the ability of the elderly to live independently.[26] With stronger muscles and bones, some old people, perhaps many, might be better able to avoid falls and broken bones, to continue to do household chores for themselves, and perhaps even to survive such acute illnesses as pneumonia. Not only would their lives be better; they might need fewer home and medical services and might spend less time in nursing homes. As important and attractive as these possibilities are, there is no good evidence about their potential. No systematic studies have yet been done of exercise for the elderly to discover how often it can make a difference, how much of a difference, and whether it can postpone or reduce dependency.

Risks

Like other preventive measures, exercise has risks as well as benefits. Some of them are implicitly accounted for in studies of benefits; for example, exercise may bring on a heart attack, but the studies already

21. Young, "Exercise in the Prevention of Disease and Disability," pp. 166, 168; and Shephard, *Physical Activity and Aging,* pp. 265–66.

22. Shephard, *Physical Activity and Aging,* pp. 248–52.

23. Young, "Exercise in the Prevention of Disease and Disability," p. 167; and Thomas and others, *Exercise and Health,* chap. 4.

24. Bjørn Krølner and others, "Physical Exercise as Prophylaxis against Involutional Vertebral Bone Loss: A Controlled Trial," *Clinical Science,* vol. 64 (May 1983), pp. 541–46; and Young, "Exercise in the Prevention of Disease and Disability," pp. 167–68. Only weight-bearing exercise strengthens bones.

25. Thomas and others, *Exercise and Health,* chap. 4; Melvin J. Stern and Patricia Cleary, "National Exercise and Heart Disease Project: Psychosocial Changes Observed during a Low-Level Exercise Program," *Archives of Internal Medicine,* vol. 141 (October 1981), pp. 1463–67; and Young, "Exercise in the Prevention of Disease and Disability," pp. 163, 167.

26. Young, "Exercise in the Prevention of Disease and Disability," p. 162; and Shephard, *Physical Activity and Aging,* pp. 286–91.

discussed show that this risk is far outweighed by the benefits, and the net effect is fewer heart attacks.[27] Many risks, however, are not caught in this way. The most obvious is the risk of injury. Exercise, especially its more vigorous forms, is responsible for broken bones, strains, sprains, and inflammation of the tendons and other structures around the joints.

Two studies of running demonstrate that the risks of this form of exercise can be substantial. One of them reviewed the experience of more than 1,000 runners who participated in a race in Atlanta.[28] During the following year, more than a third of those who continued to run or jog at least six miles a week suffered an injury serious enough to persuade them to cut back on running for a while. The knee and foot were the most common sites of injury. Not all the hazards were due to the exercise: dog bites and collisions with bicycles or cars were recorded, and a surprisingly large number of runners—more than 7 percent—had things thrown at them by people along the route. Fifteen percent of the runners consulted a doctor about their injuries.

Injuries can be much more frequent during something as strenuous as a marathon. A study of a British marathon found that 18 percent of those who tried to run the full distance (a half-marathon was run at the same time) stopped for help at the first aid stations along the way.[29] Stiffness, cramp, and torn muscles or ligaments were the most common problems; blisters and chafing were next. Of 2,289 full-marathon runners, 26 were sent to the hospital, although only 4 had to remain there overnight.

Some of these injuries could be avoided with better training, better equipment, and more care to increase the amount of exercise slowly and gradually. Children need special attention because they are particularly vulnerable to injury during periods of rapid growth.[30] But some risk will inevitably remain. As yet, not much is known about how extensive that risk is in the general population of exercisers. Even less is known about possible long-term risks, especially to joints, from the injuries and lesser

27. Thomas and others, *Exercise and Health*; and David S. Siscovick and others, "The Incidence of Primary Cardiac Arrest during Vigorous Exercise," *New England Journal of Medicine*, vol. 311 (October 4, 1984), pp. 874–77.

28. Jeffrey P. Koplan and others, "An Epidemiologic Study of the Benefits and Risks of Running," *Journal of the American Medical Association*, vol. 248 (December 17, 1982), pp. 3118–21.

29. J. P. Nicholl and B. T. Williams, "Injuries Sustained by Runners during a Popular Marathon," *British Journal of Sports Medicine*, vol. 17 (March 1983), pp. 10–15.

30. Lyle J. Micheli, "Overuse Injuries in Children's Sports: The Growth Factor," *Orthopedic Clinics of North America*, vol. 14 (April 1983), pp. 340–43.

stresses that are part of exercise. The exercise boom in many countries indicates the need to learn more about the risks as well as the benefits and, at the same time, presents an opportunity to study this natural experiment. Several authors have urged that the opportunity be used to do studies of large populations.[31]

Costs of Exercise—The Evidence

In the fall of 1978 the American College of Sports Medicine published guidelines for exercise that have been widely accepted.[32] By prescribing frequency and time, they provide a starting point for considering costs. The college recommended that to improve fitness, particularly the fitness of the heart and lungs, healthy adults should exercise three to five times a week, for fifteen to sixty minutes at a time. The exercise should be reasonably intense, requiring not less than 60 percent of an individual's maximum heart rate nor more than 90 percent (the maximum heart rate is approximately 220 minus the individual's age). The kind of exercise is not particularly important as long as it uses large muscle groups and can be maintained at the recommended level of intensity, although the discussion accompanying the guidelines points out that running and jumping activities are associated with more injuries for beginners than are other types of exercise. It also notes that older people need to take longer to reach the recommended level of exercise.

The college made it plain that it had produced the guidelines, not because all the evidence was in, but because exercise was becoming so popular that some sort of guidelines were badly needed. It reviewed a great deal of research before reaching its conclusions. This research does not link exercise directly to improvements in health, but to intermediate measures, particularly maximum oxygen intake (a good indicator of the condition of the cardiovascular system), weight, and body composition (fat and lean). The recommended level of exercise is designed to improve fitness significantly in all three dimensions. If

31. Koplan and others, "Epidemiologic Study of the Benefits and Risks of Running"; and "Symposium: Exercise, Health, and Medicine," *The Lancet* (May 21, 1983), p. 1171.

32. American College of Sports Medicine, "Position Statement on the Recommended Quantity and Quality of Exercise for Developing and Maintaining Fitness in Healthy Adults" (Indianapolis, Ind.: ACSM, Fall 1978).

cardiovascular fitness is the primary concern, ten to fifteen minutes of exercise at a time is enough to produce a significant improvement.

Considerable uncertainty remains about the amount and kind of exercise necessary to achieve the benefits reported from studies of heart disease and other conditions. It is unlikely that a single, optimum level of exercise exists, since different kinds of exercise produce different benefits. And again, there is no evidence from randomized, controlled trials that now-sedentary individuals who do not have heart disease can reduce their risk of acquiring it by taking up exercise; the published studies compare already active people with sedentary people.[33] Indeed, not everyone believes that the case has been made for strenuous exercise for adults. One researcher, for example, argues that, while the case for moderate exercise is strong, further research should be done before urging adults to take up strenuous exercise.[34]

Expenses of an Exercise Program

The financial outlays associated with exercise can vary a great deal depending on an individual's interests and motivation. A determined person who is not particularly interested in sports can meet the guidelines of the American College of Sports Medicine by exercising at home, doing calisthenics and running in place or jumping rope. Or a home program can be supplemented by walking or jogging around the neighborhood. The costs in this case are minimal—some suitable clothing, good shoes for walking or running, soap and water for extra showers and laundry, a little extra wear and tear on the house, and perhaps an exercise book or two. Some people might add an exercise mat, small weights, or other accessories. If the individual is careful and avoids any need to visit a doctor for injuries, costs for the first year might amount to $100 to $200, dropping to less than $100 a year after that—for new shoes and clothes as necessary, the soap and water, and so on.

Most people, however, prefer the companionship, guidance, and challenge provided by organized or competitive forms of exercise— aerobics, swimming, tennis, or basketball, for example. Such activities call for more resources: special facilities, equipment, perhaps a professional leader or teacher; certainly someone must oversee the use and

33. Rigotti and others, "Exercise and Coronary Heart Disease"; and Haskell and Blair, "Physical Activity Component," p. 110.
34. Holloszy, "Exercise, Health, and Aging," p. 2.

maintenance of the facility. There may be transportation costs as well—gas, depreciation, and parking fees, or charges for public transportation. The outlays quickly surpass those for exercise at home.

A cost-effectiveness analysis of exercise requires estimates of these costs to link with the probable benefits, estimates representative of the activities of a large group of people with different tastes and needs. Ideally, the estimates will be made in enough detail to permit their combination for the analysis of different populations, or their separation for the analysis of subgroups. No such estimates have been published and this discussion will not attempt to create them. Instead, its purpose is to describe the range of costs that should be included, especially those items that are often overlooked, and to suggest the size of some of them from the fragmentary evidence in the literature.

One alternative to the go-it-alone exercise plan is an exercise program at work. Workplace programs have received considerable attention in the literature and some authors contend they have special advantages.[35] When the facility is in the same building, convenience is a major advantage. And the program can make use of existing staff newsletters and the like for publicity. An obvious limitation is that only fairly large employers can afford to provide an on-site program. But by the same token a large employer can produce enough participants to keep the cost per person reasonable.

Although few authors give cost estimates for workplace programs, most agree on the kinds of resources required.[36] They note the importance of a trained leader, at least part-time if not full-time, who may be assisted by other professional staff, or by amateurs from among the company's employees. At a minimum, facilities should include an exercise room with some equipment, and space for changing and showering. The facilities can be much more elaborate; some companies provide everything from racquetball courts to a swimming pool in addition to space for individual and group exercises.

One expert has estimated the following costs for workplace programs

35. Roy J. Shephard, "Employee Health and Fitness: The State of the Art," *Preventive Medicine*, vol. 12, no. 5 (1983), pp. 644–53; and Haskell and Blair, "Physical Activity Component."

36. Shephard, "Employee Health and Fitness," pp. 647–48; Haskell and Blair, "Physical Activity Component," pp. 115–16; Robert C. Cantu, ed., *The Exercising Adult* (Lexington, Mass.: Collamore Press, 1982); and Jonathan E. Fielding, "Effectiveness of Employee Health Improvement Programs," *Journal of Occupational Medicine*, vol. 24 (November 1982), p. 912.

of the most basic kind.[37] The costs are the average for one participant for one year.

Number of participants	Facility	Cost (1982 $)
5–50	Minimal facility, testing, and exercise prescription	100–350
75–250	150-to-300-square-meter facility, part-time or full-time supervisor	250–350
400–850	600-to-1,200-square-meter facility, full-time supervisor	200–350

These estimates include only some of the expenditures for an exercise program—some professional help, and amortization of the investment required to renovate space for the new purpose. They appear to omit the employer's outlay for the space itself, which involves rental or depreciation and overhead expenses; the cost of utilities; and the cost of the time of regular employees who volunteer to help with the program. And they omit the costs incurred by employees for clothing and equipment. The brief descriptions indicate that the estimates do include the costs of basic testing to help set the appropriate level of exercise and measure progress.

Medical Care Expenses

There is a wide range of opinion about testing—particularly about whether people should be examined by a doctor before they begin to exercise, and how extensive that exam should be. The choice of policy can have a big impact on the costs of exercise.

In several of its publications, the American Heart Association recommends that everyone should be evaluated by a physician before taking up exercise or increasing it significantly.[38] For people known to have heart disease, and those in whom heart disease is suspected, the association also recommends an exercise test;[39] during an exercise test,

37. Shephard, "Employee Health and Fitness," p. 648.

38. American Heart Association Committee on Exercise, *Exercise Testing and Training of Apparently Healthy Individuals: A Handbook for Physicians* (New York: The Association, 1972); and American Heart Association, *The Exercise Standards Book* (The Association, June 1979), p. 45.

39. American Heart Association, *Exercise Standards Book*, p. 45. Exercise tests involve some risk—one death and three nonfatal complications occur for every 10,000 tests. See Thomas and others, *Exercise and Health*, chap. 6; and American Heart Association Committee on Exercise, *Exercise Testing*, p. 3. There is considerable controversy over whether exercise tests are reliable enough as a test for heart problems to be worth doing. See, for example, Henry A. Solomon, *The Exercise Myth* (Harcourt Brace Jovanovich, 1984), pp. 34–37.

the patient runs on a treadmill, pedals a stationary bicycle, or performs some other activity while the physician measures the response of the heart and blood pressure. In several booklets aimed at patients rather than physicians, the association gives a somewhat more selective set of guidelines, advising sedentary men over 45 and sedentary women over 50, as well as anyone with heart disease, hypertension, or other symptoms or conditions that might indicate special problems, to consult a doctor before beginning an exercise program.[40]

Another group of experts, Thomas and his colleagues, favor the more selective approach.[41] They note with approval a Canadian program that uses a list of seven questions to let people decide for themselves whether they should see a doctor before plunging into an exercise regimen. The questions focus on heart disease, but they also ask about joint problems and age—being over 65 and sedentary is, by itself, enough to indicate that a medical examination is a good idea. In early tests, the questions prompted fewer than half of all adults to see a doctor, although still somewhat more than really needed to.

In Great Britain, the Royal College of Physicians of London and the British Cardiac Society have agreed on a recommendation that minimizes the use of special evaluations, arguing that "most people do not need a medical examination before starting an exercise programme" as long as the workout begins at a low level and builds intensity very slowly.[42] They suggest seeking medical advice only if unexpected symptoms develop.

For people who already have cardiovascular disease, Thomas and his colleagues recommend not only an initial evaluation by a doctor but participation in a medically supervised program of exercise. They add that a medically supervised program is also desirable, although not mandatory, for people at high risk for cardiovascular disease. And for everyone, they believe that periodic visits to a physician can be useful to help maintain motivation as well as for advice and care.

Partly offsetting the costs, medical and otherwise, of an exercise

40. "Exercise Diary"; "Swimming for a Healthy Heart"; "Dancing for a Healthy Heart"; "Walking for a Healthy Heart"; and "Running for a Healthy Heart." All of these American Heart Association pamphlets were published in Dallas during 1984. The symptoms and conditions include frequent pain in the chest or arm after exercise, extreme breathlessness after mild exercise, dizzy spells, bone or joint problems, and diabetes.
41. Thomas and others, *Exercise and Health*, chap. 5.
42. "Symposium: Exercise, Health and Medicine," p. 1171.

program are the potential savings in medical costs due to less heart disease. Additional savings will accrue if regular exercise makes it possible for the elderly to continue to live independently when they would otherwise require help at home or even transfer to a nursing home. There may even be recreational savings analogous to those in medical care—if they could be estimated, the costs of whatever people would do if they were not exercising could be subtracted from the costs of exercise.

Time

One resource that needs to enter discussions of cost is the exerciser's time. Understandably, the costs usually considered are those that involve actual outlays of cash. No one pays for an exerciser's time, but it is nonetheless a real resource. Time used to exercise cannot be used to do other things. The pressure of time is one reason that people give up exercising, and it also influences the kind of exercise they choose. Although time is involved in any prevention program, ignoring it may not distort the results of an evaluation when the total time required is small, as it is, for example, for one-time vaccinations. But so much time is required by exercise that its omission from an evaluation would be an important distortion.

At a minimum, the time required is the fifteen to sixty minutes three to five times a week that the American College of Sports Medicine recommends. Add to that any travel time and the time to prepare for exercising and to shower and change afterwards. Organized sports can involve even more time, particularly for parents who are called on to transport children to games and help run local sports activities. The time used by exercise is a major resource cost. How to represent that cost in a cost-effectiveness evaluation is taken up in the next section.

Putting the Pieces Together

The evidence about the health effects and costs of exercise has been outlined. The next stage in a cost-effectiveness analysis is to combine the evidence to estimate aggregate effects and costs. This section describes the steps involved in developing aggregate estimates, both to explain the procedures appropriate to the case of exercise and to complete the discussion of the principles of cost-effectiveness analysis begun in chapters 2 and 3.

The cost-effectiveness evaluation outlined here considers exercise as a way to improve health, as did the evaluations of measles vaccine and of screening and treatment for hypertension presented in chapters 2 and 3.[43] The section has four parts: (1) how to choose the perspective of a proposed study, (2) how to combine the information about health effects, (3) how to combine the information about costs, and (4) how to present the aggregate estimates to help people draw conclusions about the cost-effectiveness of exercise.

Determining a Perspective

The first issue in any evaluation is whether it should reflect the point of view of the entire society, of a government program, of an employer, or of an individual. The health effects and costs that should be included will differ according to the perspective chosen.

An analysis conducted from the social perspective aims at calculating the net gain in health and the net use of resources for society as a whole. The evaluations of measles vaccine and hypertension treatment chose the social perspective. Both analyses included gains in health net of any losses, regardless of who enjoyed the gains or suffered the losses; and they included costs net of savings, regardless of who incurred the costs or pocketed the savings. For example, the study of measles vaccine counted only the cost of institutionalization and special education over and above the cost of care for a normal child—the rest of the cost was offset by savings elsewhere in society. Similarly, savings in medical costs were subtracted from the costs of vaccination and of hypertension treatment, although the people who made the outlays might not see the savings.

A director of a government program, an employer, or an individual will often consider only the narrower set of effects and costs that applies

43. Once exercise, or any preventive measure, has been shown to bring a reasonable return in health for the expenditure—to be cost-effective—the next issue is whether public or private institutions can usefully help to promote it. Cost-effectiveness analysis can also be applied to methods of promotion. This section concentrates on the cost-effectiveness of exercise itself rather than of the promotion of exercise because the first issue logically precedes the second. But that emphasis should not be interpreted to mean that promotional policies are unimportant, or that they do not need to be evaluated.

to him or her. For example, although medicare might save money for medicaid by paying for a service that reduced the need for nursing homes, the saving would not appear in an analysis that calculated cost-effectiveness strictly from the point of view of the medicare program. Similarly, if a program undertaken at the workplace postponed illness until most employees had retired, an analysis done from the employer's point of view would count the savings to the employer, but not the extra costs to medicare.

These examples help explain why the social point of view is the logical perspective for questions of public policy and the one that appears most frequently in the published literature. It is the only point of view that never counts as a gain what is really someone else's loss. Program directors, employers, and others sometimes use this perspective as well, even when their direct interests are narrower, because they want to know what effect their choices will have on the larger society. They would, of course, like to point to any gains that accrue to the rest of society, but they should also count any losses.

The discussion that follows assumes that exercise is being evaluated from the social point of view first—that is, all costs and benefits are considered—and only secondarily, if at all, from narrower perspectives. It is somewhat more difficult to design an analysis so that all major perspectives can be evaluated. It requires, for example, not only that total medical costs and savings be estimated but that they be broken down according to the specific group that pays or receives them. Similarly, health effects must be assigned to the right group. Some of this accounting detail is generated anyway in the process of producing aggregate estimates, but not all of it.

For the social perspective, the entire population in the area covered by the policy constitutes the relevant population. The measles vaccine and hypertension treatment studies applied to the population of the United States, but if either had covered only a state or community, the population of that area would have been the right base for the analysis. The total population should be broken down into subgroups if it is known that some of them have benefits, risks, or costs very different from others. The additional detail makes it possible to calculate cost-effectiveness for the various groups and for alternative policies that might affect them differently—for example, a policy aimed at inducing people at high risk for heart disease to exercise regularly.

Representing Health Effects

To represent the gains in health from exercise, all the principal health effects—good and bad—must be estimated for all the major groups in society. It is then extremely helpful to translate them into a single measure of health outcome. Exploring the implications of the health gains for absenteeism, turnover, school attendance, and other activities may also be important for some analyses.

Ideally, estimates of the health gains from exercise would come from a large, well-designed clinical trial based on a representative sample of the population. This trial would compare people who engaged in different amounts of exercise with people who continued to lead sedentary lives and would report differences in overall death rates, regardless of cause, in sickness, and in injuries among the groups. From this information the gains in health to be expected if the entire population took up exercise could be calculated. The obstacles to such a trial are formidable, however, not to mention the expense; one attempt to conduct a national trial in the United States was abandoned after a preliminary study showed that the dropout rate would be extremely high.[44]

The more pragmatic alternative for most cost-effectiveness analyses, and in many cases the only alternative, is to build estimates from the fragmentary evidence of a number of studies already at hand, filling in any gaps with reasonable guesses. When data are plentiful, this process can produce reliable estimates at considerably less cost than a clinical trial.

The process can be very simple or very complicated. The evaluation of measles vaccine, for example, used statistics on deaths and retardation from measles to estimate the health gains from the vaccine; the authors simplified their task by ignoring the side effects of the vaccine and by making no attempt to measure other possible health effects from measles—for example, learning disabilities less serious than retardation—although they did estimate days lost from school and work. In their study of hypertension, Weinstein and Stason used data from the Framingham study that showed deaths and sickness from heart disease according to level of blood pressure; in order to estimate the gains in health from lowering blood pressure, they developed several alternative sets of

44. Rigotti and others, "Exercise and Coronary Heart Disease," p. 398.

assumptions about how far hypertension could be reduced, to what extent treatment could produce the same health as naturally low pressures, and how long it took for maximum effect to be achieved—aspects of treatment about which knowledge is still incomplete. The procedures involved in Eddy's evaluations of cancer screening were more complicated still, requiring sophisticated models of the disease process, built up piece by piece from different studies, to show the gain from catching a cancer earlier rather than later.

The information available about exercise is sufficient to support an estimating process of this kind. The best studies of the relation between exercise and heart disease among middle-aged men provide a good foundation. They show the size of the effect and the shape of the relation—heart disease declines steadily as exercise increases, and the effect is greater if the exercise is vigorous—and show them, moreover, for an important disease in an important group. To complete the calculations for this group, injuries from exercise and the effect of exercise on deaths and illness from other causes must be estimated. The simplest assumption is that all other good and bad effects roughly cancel so that only heart disease matters.

For other sex and age groups, the more limited direct evidence can be combined with some of the general insights provided by the studies of middle-aged men. For example, where there is no direct evidence on the subject, one possible approach is to assume that the relation between exercise and heart disease has the same shape for other groups as it does for middle-aged men—that is, heart disease declines steadily with more exercise for women and for younger and older men also, and vigorous exercise is especially effective. Reasonable estimates of the size of the effect, as opposed to the general shape of the relation, may be available directly from studies of these groups; or it may be possible to derive estimates by, for example, piecing together information from studies of the effect of exercise on maximum oxygen intake in these groups with information on the link between maximum oxygen intake and heart disease in middle-aged men.

A particular difficulty for the estimation process is the uncertainty about the true effect of exercise on heart disease. The true effect lies somewhere between the gain shown when other risk factors for heart disease are ignored and the gain after correction for them. The conservative approach would be to use the lower estimate—the estimate after correction for other risk factors. Or both alternatives could be evaluated to see how great the difference is.

The end result is a series of estimates showing the various gains and losses in health for the entire population and for subgroups of particular interest. These can include changes in deaths from all causes, in deaths from heart disease, in nonfatal heart attacks and episodes of chest pain, in leg and foot injuries, and so on. Unfortunately, the evidence gives out altogether on many long-term effects—most studies have been of rather short duration, and some of the potential long-term risks of exercise have not yet been documented.

Once the health effects have been expressed in numbers of lives saved, injuries suffered, and so on, it is helpful—at times essential—to translate them into a common unit in order to arrive at an overall assessment. The year of healthy life, or quality-adjusted life-year, discussed in chapter 3, provides a reasonable and workable unit. For example, a runner with a permanently stiff ankle might be willing to give up .05 of a year to live the remaining .95 of the year without the disability; the value of the year with the stiff ankle would then be .95 of a healthy year. Similarly, someone suffering from frequent chest pain might value a year in that state at .80 of a healthy year. With something like exercise, which can have so many different effects on health, the methods developed for valuing states of health discussed in chapter 3 are particularly appropriate.[45] When the state does not last a year, but only a few days or weeks, the value for a year can be built up from the value for each day or week that goes into it.[46]

After translation into years of healthy life gained or lost, the health effects can be added to arrive at the net gain in healthy life. This is a useful summary for even a single policy when there are many kinds

45. These methods are described in Robert M. Kaplan, "Quality of Life Measurement," in Paul Karoly, ed., *Measurement Strategies in Health Psychology* (Wiley, 1985), pp. 115–46; and Marilyn Bergner and others, "The Sickness Impact Profile: Development and Final Revision of a Health Status Measure," *Medical Care,* vol. 19 (August 1981), pp. 787–805.

46. The case of exercise brings up the intriguing possibility that a year of healthy life may not be a fixed state. Exercise makes some people feel better than they did before they exercised, even though they were not aware of any symptoms or disability in their earlier state. Thus they might value a year of healthy life with regular exercise more highly than a year of healthy but sedentary life. Researchers who use health status indexes are aware of this possibility and some would take it into account by allowing values greater than 1.0 for a healthy year.

of health effects. It is essential for comparing very different programs. The issues of summarization and comparison are discussed at greater length later in this chapter and in chapter 5.

A further kind of translation can be useful in some evaluations—the translation of health effects into their consequences for productive activities. More years of life usually mean more years of paid or unpaid work for adults and more years of schooling for children. Several studies—most of them unfortunately not well designed and thus not very reliable—have found that exercise is associated with less absenteeism and turnover, outcomes of particular interest to employers.[47] The important point is that these outcomes are not in addition to the health effects, but are the consequences of those effects. As argued in chapter 2, consequences such as future earnings due to lives saved can legitimately be presented as supplementary detail about the health effects, but not as benefits over and above those effects.

Representing Costs

It is helpful to think of the costs of exercise as falling into two general categories—the costs incurred by people committed to regular exercise, and the costs of persuading people to exercise. The discussion of costs earlier in this chapter dealt mostly with the first kind of costs, although the distinction is not always hard and fast; providing more convenient facilities and more appealing forms of exercise is as much a part of persuasion as are counseling sessions or posters. Costs can differ among individuals depending on their special requirements as well as on the difficulty of convincing them to stay with a regular program. For example, someone who has survived a heart attack may be highly motivated but probably needs a medically supervised program, which adds to expenditures. Someone else, for whom unsupervised exercise is appropriate, may be so disinclined to exercise, or so busy, that large sums are required to persuade the person to begin, or to make exercise more convenient.

If the ideal clinical trial were carried out to measure the health effects of exercise, most of the costs could be measured at the same time.[48] In

---

47. Fielding, "Effectiveness of Employee Health Improvement Programs," p. 910.

48. Drummond and Stoddart have discussed the conditions in which it makes sense to evaluate costs as well as health effects in a clinical trial. Michael F. Drummond and Greg L. Stoddart, "Economic Analysis and Clinical Trials," *Controlled Clinical Trials*, vol. 5 (June 1984), pp. 115–28.

principle at least, both kinds of costs—those of exercise and those of persuasion—could be measured by evaluating groups that required different amounts of persuasion and special care.

In practice, costs must usually be pieced together from unrelated sources of information to an even greater extent than health effects. There have been no studies of the costs of exercise to match those of its health effects in care, accuracy, or generality. To begin the piecing process, the analyst might start with the kinds of exercise people currently engage in, then crudely estimate the actual costs for each kind using available data on the retail prices of equipment, membership fees for various facilities, and so on.[49] The estimates of health effects are themselves another valuable source of information, since they indicate how often, and for what diseases, savings in medical costs can be expected, and how often, and for what conditions, the side effects of exercise will involve expense over and above the costs of exercise itself.

The time required to exercise is a true cost but difficult to value in dollar terms so that it can be added to other costs. For people with paying jobs, one possibility is to price their time at their hourly wage, and this approach is sometimes used in cost-effectiveness studies. Even for paid workers, this method of valuation is subject to a number of criticisms, and for people who are not paid—children, retirees, homemakers—it is not practical.

The basic stumbling block is that the appropriate value is not a wage rate but the value an individual actually places on that time.[50] As for any cost, the fundamental concept to be measured is the opportunity cost— the payment required to persuade the owner of a resource to make it available. The difference is that there is no market for leisure time and so no way to observe a market price for this resource. Further, the value of time depends on whose time it is, just as the value of land depends on its location, so there is no reason to expect the price to be the same for everyone. For someone who dislikes exercise and is under pressure to do a great many other things, the time spent exercising represents a substantial cost. For someone who loves exercise for itself, the time spent represents a very small cost, no matter how many other activities compete for that time. After considering the same problem in studies of

49. It is easier to estimate the minimum cost of exercise, supposing people were willing to follow such a program, than to estimate the costs necessary to induce them to exercise.

50. E. J. Mishan, *Cost-Benefit Analysis* (Praeger, 1976), chap. 41.

transportation—the time taken or saved by different forms of transport—one analyst concluded that there is no single, correct way to value time.

What cannot be valued is too often ignored. These problems should not be allowed to push time out of the evaluation. There are two practical possibilities and the analyst can use either or both in the same analysis. Certainly, an attempt should be made to estimate the amount of time used in exercise, even if the estimate must be rough and even if no dollar value is put on it. The analyst can then conclude that exercise brings so many extra years of healthy life in return for so much expenditure[51] and so much time on the part of the exercisers themselves. In addition, accepting the shortcomings of the estimate, the analyst might put a dollar value on time simply to indicate its importance relative to other costs. The average wage would be a reasonable value for this purpose, especially for an analysis of adult exercisers.

Presenting the Results

An evaluation of exercise carried through to this point would produce an array of estimates of the health effects and costs of exercise. The major items are shown in an illustrative table shell (table 4-1). The health effects are first described in their natural units. They can also be translated into the number of healthy years gained, with gains in future years appropriately discounted, and totaled. Costs associated with different items and total costs are estimated, again with costs in future years appropriately discounted before being added together. The time spent by exercisers is also estimated, although not necessarily translated into dollar terms. The health effects and costs should be shown for subgroups of the population as well as for the population as a whole.

There are two ways to present this information to help show the balance of costs and health effects. The balance sheet, an array of information like that in table 4-1, was used in the measles vaccine study discussed in chapter 2; it retains much of the detail of the analysis. The cost-effectiveness ratio, described in chapter 3 and used in the study of hypertension treatment, is particularly useful for comparing large numbers of alternatives. To derive this ratio the total costs shown in the table shell are divided by the total years of healthy life gained; the result is the

---

51. The time of people who earn their living helping others exercise is represented in costs by their salaries.

Table 4-1. Table Shell Showing Items in a Cost-Effectiveness Evaluation of Exercise (Balance-Sheet Method of Presentation)

Health effects	In natural units	In years of healthy life gained
Years of life saved	000	000
Cases of disability prevented	000	000
Other improvements in quality of life	000	000
Less side effects	(000)	(000)
Total[a]	. . .	000

Costs	In dollars
Exercise expenses (clothes, equipment, facilities and staff, etc.)	000
Medical care expenses	
Initial evaluations, care for injuries	000
Less savings from disease prevented	(000)
Time involved in exercising	000
Total[a]	000

a. Future health effects and costs are discounted before being summed. See discussions in chapters 2 and 3.

cost per year of healthy life. The two should be viewed as supplements to each other, useful for different situations, rather than as mutually exclusive alternatives.

The value of the balance sheet is exactly that it does show so much detail. The reader of the balance sheet can see what particular gains in health make up the total, how much comes from extra years of life and how much from better health, and which groups in the population benefit especially. Similarly, the sources of cost can be presented in detail and the time spent by exercisers can be shown separately, without a dollar valuation. The balance sheet can include additional detail on the conse-quences of the health effects if these are of interest—earnings, absentee-ism, days in school, days in hospitals or nursing homes, and so on. The detail gives the user a good sense of what the proposed program is about in terms that most people can readily understand. Because of this advantage, the Office of Technology Assessment in the U.S. Congress and the participants in a symposium on prevention sponsored by the Ciba Foundation both recommended this method of presentation.[52]

The disadvantage of the balance sheet is that it is a cumbersome way

52. Office of Technology Assessment, *Strategies for Medical Technology Assessment* (Government Printing Office, 1982), p. 61; and Ciba Foundation, *Value of Preventive Medicine*, Symposium 110 (London: Pitman, 1985), pp. 84, 187, 215.

to compare alternatives, and comparisons are a major purpose of cost-effectiveness analysis. For some comparisons, the detail is unnecessary because only one item will change; for example, balance sheets showing the results for two policies toward medical evaluation will differ only in the estimate for medical costs. For others, the detail is overwhelming because the balance sheets may differ in nearly every item—in a comparison between measles vaccine for children and exercise for adults, for example.

The value of the cost-effectiveness ratio is that it makes comparisons easy. For each alternative, all health effects are reduced to one number, the gain in years of healthy life. Costs are expressed as a total number of dollars. The cost-effectiveness ratio—the cost per year of healthy life—can then be compared across any number of alternatives, because the same units are used for each. At the same time, whenever the cost-effectiveness ratio seems too much of a summary, the user can refer to the balance sheet for the alternative in question to find out more about what went into the ratio. The ratio and balance sheet complement each other, each supplying what the other lacks.

This chapter has suggested many comparisons that the analyst might want to explore in an evaluation of exercise.

—Size of effect. The cost-effectiveness of exercise can be calculated for two extreme cases: (1) exercise is responsible for the entire reduction in heart disease associated with it, or (2) it is responsible for only the reduction left after correction for other risk factors. Exercise will clearly be more cost-effective in the first case, but only the calculations can show how much more.

—Medical policies. The recommendation that all adults receive physicals before beginning exercise can be compared with more selective policies. Different policies will clearly affect costs and may affect benefits.

—Subgroups. The cost-effectiveness of exercise for different subgroups of the population can be calculated. The ratios will reflect differences in health effects, risks, and costs among the groups.

—Perspectives. Cost-effectiveness ratios can be calculated from the point of view of the individual, of employers, and of certain government programs, as well as from the social point of view.

—Medical costs in added years. It was noted in chapter 2 that medical costs in years of life saved by a preventive measure should only be included when the issue is the measure's potential effect on total medical expenditures, not when the point of the analysis is to determine whether it is a good investment. Nonetheless, the current interest in the narrower issue—and especially in whether prevention can cut medical expenditures—makes it worth analyzing.

An analysis can also extend beyond these comparisons to include the evaluation of alternative policies for persuading people to exercise. Persuasion can take the form of promotional activities such as advertising, better or more convenient exercise facilities, subsidies for the cost of facilities, time off from work to exercise, and so on. Each alternative will persuade additional people to exercise but at additional cost. The analysis will require information about how many additional people and what additional cost in order to produce cost-effectiveness ratios that will show which methods work best.

In addition to the cost-effectiveness estimates themselves, the degree of uncertainty associated with those estimates needs to be emphasized in the presentation of the results. Regardless of how the results are presented—whether in the form of a balance sheet or a cost-effectiveness ratio—they are subject to uncertainty. This uncertainty is hinted at by the ratios calculated for alternative assumptions about health effects and costs, but even these leave the user with the impression that, under the circumstances specified, the cost-effectiveness of exercise (or hypertension treatment or measles vaccination) is a certain number when, in fact, it is somewhere in the general neighborhood of that number. In some cases, when the available information is thin and not very reliable, the general neighborhood may be quite large.

It is desirable to attach a measure of uncertainty to each estimate, such as the standard deviations that are calculated for estimates derived from sample surveys. Since much of the information used in evaluations does not come from sample surveys, the direct calculation of standard deviations is not possible. One expert has proposed an alternative approach.[53] He suggests that the analyst ask experts to indicate the likely values for important variables—not just the average but the values they would consider the largest or smallest possible, or some narrower boundaries. The analyst can then assign an approximate statistical distribution to each variable, generate dozens, or hundreds, of estimates of the cost-effectiveness ratio under a given set of conditions, and from these calculate both an average estimate and a standard deviation.

53. Mishan, *Cost-Benefit Analysis*, chap. 56.

Some Further Issues

Like vaccines or screening tests, changes in lifestyle share some characteristics but no two of them are exactly the same. Each one must be evaluated separately. If programs to keep people from smoking are a good investment in health, it does not automatically follow that programs to encourage them to exercise or change their diet will be. This section brings out some additional similarities and differences that shape the results of an evaluation. The discussion is organized around the factors that have been used throughout this study—populations and frequency, risk, uncertainty, individual values, and time.

Perhaps the outstanding feature of preventive measures that work through lifestyle is their *frequency*—they involve everyday habits that can take considerable time. Like many other preventive measures, they can apply to large *populations*, often the entire population, but it is this dailiness that distinguishes them. Small costs and small discomforts build up quickly when they are repeated often. For example, an individual who devotes an hour three times a week to exercise—thirty minutes for the exercise itself, and thirty minutes for changing, showering, and traveling—spends almost twenty working days on exercise in the course of the year.

Changes in lifestyle are often proposed for everyone, as though everyone were at equal *risk* of disease, but this may not always be the case. It may be possible to identify groups at particularly high risk for some aspects of lifestyle and to tailor changes more specifically to those risks. Diet is an area where further investigation may show that different groups need different guidelines. Not everyone appears to react the same way to salt, for example, and some people have serious allergies to important foods, such as milk. One researcher examined a more selective approach of this kind when she evaluated a change in diet, not for all 10-year-old boys, but only for those found to be at the highest extreme of the cholesterol distribution.[54]

Changes in lifestyle can themselves entail important risks. This point is often overlooked and changes in everyday habits are sometimes discussed as though they were entirely without risk. Clearly exercise

---

54. Shan Cretin, "Cost/Benefit Analysis of Treatment and Prevention of Myocardial Infarction," *Health Services Research*, vol. 12 (Summer 1977), pp. 174–89.

can cause injuries in the short run and may prove to cause long-run problems as well. More generally, not much is known about the risks of changes in the many personal habits that constitute lifestyle; the dearth of information undoubtedly contributes to the tendency to believe they are insignificant. The problem is compounded because so many studies look at the link between some aspect of lifestyle and a single disease— an approach that is useful for developing hypotheses, but which cannot show the overall effect of the habit. For example, low levels of cholesterol are associated with low death rates from heart disease, but they are also associated with a somewhat greater risk of cancer.[55]

The lack of knowledge about risks argues for caution. *Uncertainty* because of lack of information is a problem for any kind of medical care, but it particularly weighs against sudden change in the area of prevention. In part, this reflects the differences in populations and in time. Prevention puts more people at risk, earlier, than does acute care and it is correspondingly more important to be sure that the magnitude of that risk lies within reasonable bounds. It also reflects the difference in the initial positions of the people to be treated. Consider the extreme case. Most people agree that it is reasonable and ethical to try an unproven therapy on a dying patient; the patient has little to lose. The person considering prevention, who is healthy and apparently, or in truth, free of disease, has a great deal to lose. Thus it is reasonable to be more cautious about adopting a preventive measure than about acute care.

Time and *individual values* play their usual parts. The health benefits of changes in lifestyle, at least the chief ones, come rather late in life. Any costs of those changes start much earlier and continue throughout life. Not everyone will weigh those costs and benefits the same way. For some, particularly those who do not begrudge the time required, the benefits are ample repayment for the costs and they include the immediate pleasure of the activity as well as its long-term effects on health. Others prefer the pleasures and convenience of less healthy lifestyles.

Many people have already decided that the costs and benefits of a change in lifestyle look worthwhile to them. The last two decades have seen major changes in living habits—regular exercise, low-fat diets, an emphasis on fruits and vegetables, and smoking-cessation programs are becoming part of the common culture.[56] These trends in themselves can

55. "Mass Strategies of Prevention—The Swings and Roundabouts," *The Lancet* (December 4, 1982), p. 1257.
56. See, for example, Weldon J. Walker, "Changing U.S. Life Style and Declining

change the balance of costs and benefits for others. As more people disapprove of smoking and try to restrict it, smoking becomes less pleasant and more difficult for those who continue. As more people take up exercise, it becomes the thing to do. Individual values change with the times.

The case of lifestyle underscores the point that the principal consideration in thinking about an investment in health is total cost, not the cost in any particular sector of the economy. Many of the costs of lifestyle changes occur outside the medical sector. In some cases, a change in lifestyle may reduce costs in the medical sector, in others it may not. But a saving in the medical sector is not much of a gain to society if it is the result of larger expenditures elsewhere. Nor is added medical expenditure of much concern if it is offset by savings elsewhere. The sensible approach is to look at the total costs required by a preventive measure, wherever those costs occur, and to compare them with the improvements in health they produce.

Vascular Mortality—A Retrospective," *New England Journal of Medicine*, vol. 308 (March 17, 1983), pp. 649–51; Kenneth E. Warner, "The Effects of the Anti-Smoking Campaign on Cigarette Consumption," *American Journal of Public Health*, vol. 67 (July 1977), pp. 645–50; and Warner and Hillary A. Murt, "Impact of the Antismoking Campaign on Smoking Prevalence: A Cohort Analysis," *Journal of Public Health Policy*, vol. 3 (December 1982), pp. 374–90.

chapter five Evaluating Prevention: Some Results and a Framework for Future Studies

A growing body of research indicates that the chronic, degenerative diseases of middle and old age can often be prevented, or at least delayed many years. Advances such as new vaccines continue to be made against infectious diseases as well. These developments offer the promise of better ways to maintain health and extend life, and have caused a new surge of interest in prevention.

This study has examined the facts about some important preventive measures and the results of careful evaluations of those measures. By highlighting the full complexity of the issues, and the uniqueness of each measure, the discussions show the importance of evaluating each one individually rather than accepting generalizations about preventive measures as a group. Chapter 2 considered the smallpox and measles vaccines. Chapter 3 discussed screening tests, using screening for hypertension as the major example, and looking briefly at cancer screening. Chapter 4 described how to conduct evaluations of changes in lifestyle; the specific example in the chapter was exercise.

Conclusions

While prevention has great potential, it is neither riskless nor costless. As the preceding chapters have shown, every preventive measure involves some risk. Often the risk cannot be fully understood until the measure has been applied to large populations for a considerable time. The uncertainty fuels extended debates in scientific and policy circles. An example is the debate over smallpox vaccine, which flared again and again during two centuries, as new information, changes in the vaccine, and changes in the disease repeatedly altered the balance of benefits and risks. Once the issue is settled for one application of a measure, perhaps only temporarily, it can move on to possible new applications, as it has in the case of drug treatment for mild hypertension.

The evidence also shows that, even after allowing for savings in treatment, prevention usually adds to medical expenditures, contrary to the popular view that it reduces them. Evaluations of a number of significant preventive measures—several of which have been reviewed in this study—support this conclusion.[1] There are exceptions. For example, the Office of Technology Assessment has estimated that the vaccine against pneumococcal pneumonia might reduce medical outlays for people 45 or older, although not for younger age-groups, if the cost per person of the vaccination could be kept down through a public program.[2] But the exceptions are rare. Prevention is not the solution to the problem of rising medical expenditures.

In some cases prevention may save money in other, nonmedical, sectors of the economy.[3] Studies of the measles vaccine and of lead screening for young children both indicate that these procedures reduce expenditures for institutionalization and special education by preventing retardation among children.[4] It is not possible, however, to conclude that there are usually savings elsewhere because most analyses have not looked beyond medical expenditures. Further, the example of exercise demonstrates that some preventive steps increase expenditures outside of medical care, and that they can make substantial use of resources, such as people's time, that represent true costs but often do not appear in evaluations because no one pays for them in cash. Both possibilities—possible savings and possible costs in the rest of the economy—under-

1. For additional examples, see the reviews in Louise B. Russell, "The Economics of Prevention," in James E. Hamner III and Barbara J. Sax Jacobs, eds., *Marketing and Managing Health Care: Health Promotion and Disease Prevention* (Memphis: University of Tennessee Center for the Health Sciences, 1983), pp. 143–63; also a revised version of the same paper in *Health Policy*, vol. 4 (1984), pp. 85–100; and Donald M. Berwick, Shan Cretin, and Emmett Keeler, *Cholesterol, Children, and Heart Disease: An Analysis of Alternatives* (Oxford University Press, 1980), chap. 7.

2. Office of Technology Assessment, *A Review of Selected Federal Vaccine and Immunization Policies: Based on Case Studies of Pneumococcal Vaccine* (Government Printing Office, 1979), chap. 4.

3. Some kinds of curative care may also reduce expenditures outside the medical sector. For example, hip replacements may reduce expenditures for household help by making it possible for elderly people to remain independent.

4. Norman W. Axnick, Steven M. Shavell, and John J. Witte, "Benefits Due to Immunization against Measles," *Public Health Reports*, vol. 84 (August 1969), pp. 673–80; and Donald M. Berwick and Anthony L. Komaroff, "Cost Effectiveness of Lead Screening," *New England Journal of Medicine*, vol. 306 (June 10, 1982), pp. 1392–98.

score an important point. What really matters is not whether a preventive measure adds to costs in a particular sector, or reduces them, but the total costs it involves, wherever they occur.

These results show that prevention cannot be assumed to be a better choice than cure in every case. Individual measures must be evaluated on their merits. To date few studies have been done that attempt direct comparisons between prevention and acute care. In one of these, Cretin compared a change in diet for 10-year-old boys whose cholesterol levels were high with a policy of no prevention and intensive care for the extra heart attacks. The cost per year of life saved was somewhat less for the intensive care strategy.[5] In another, Weinstein compared drug treatment of hypertension to prevent heart disease with bypass surgery for heart disease once it occurred, the latter with and without various screening programs to identify symptomless heart disease. On the assumption that everyone adhered to the treatment regimen, the cost of screening and drug therapy for hypertension was about the same per year of life gained as the cost of bypass surgery for patients whose symptoms were obvious without special screening tests. When adherence to the drug regimen was less than perfect, bypass surgery was more cost-effective.[6] While two studies are not enough to show that prevention and cure usually produce similar results, they do reinforce the point: it cannot be assumed that prevention is invariably the better investment.

This means that choosing investments in health is more difficult than some of the claims for prevention would suggest. Sometimes prevention buys more health for the money; sometimes cure does. And indeed, since the choice must usually include some of both, the issue most often is what mix of prevention and therapy is best. It is a rare preventive measure that, like smallpox vaccine, eradicates the condition altogether; antihypertensive drugs and regular exercise, for example, substantially reduce but do not eliminate heart attacks. Curative care remains necessary for those who suffer the disease despite reasonable efforts to avoid it, as well as for those for whom prevention was introduced too late.

These conclusions challenge the most ardent supporters of preven-

5. At a discount rate of 5 percent. Shan Cretin, "Cost/Benefit Analysis of Treatment and Prevention of Myocardial Infarction," *Health Services Research*, vol. 12 (Summer 1977), pp. 184–85.

6. Milton C. Weinstein, "Economic Impact and Cost-Effectiveness of Medical Technology," paper presented at the 1981 Frank M. Norfleet Forum for the Advancement of Health, University of Tennessee Center for the Health Sciences, Memphis, Tennessee.

tion, those who claim that prevention is a path to lower medical expenditures as well as better health.[7] By insisting on both claims, the proponents have put themselves in the untenable position of arguing that a preventive measure is a good investment only if it saves money. Those less persuaded of prevention's merit then merely have to show that a measure adds to medical expenditures to stigmatize it as a bad investment.

But this logic is faulty. Without realizing it, both sides are implicitly saying that better health is not worth paying for, that it has no intrinsic value and should be approved only when it is free or, better yet, comes with a bonus in the form of savings.

Clearly good health does have intrinsic value and is worth paying for. And it does cost money. Choosing investments in prevention is thus an economic choice like any other. Prevention offers good things at some additional cost. The gains must be balanced against the costs to decide whether a particular preventive measure is a good investment.

A Framework for the Future

The question that must be asked of any preventive measure, or of any investment in health, is: are the gains in health a reasonable return for the risks and costs? That is the question cost-effectiveness analysis is designed to help answer. Like cost-benefit analysis, cost-effectiveness analysis tallies all the important gains and losses associated with a measure. Its distinguishing feature is that, unlike cost-benefit analysis, it does not put a dollar value on gains in health. Instead, these are summarized in terms of lives saved, cases of disease avoided, or when very different health effects must be combined, years of healthy life.

As part of the discussion of specific preventive measures and the evaluations that have been done of them, the preceding chapters have described the principles of cost-effectiveness analysis. Chapter 2 defined the method and gave an example of the balance-sheet approach to displaying the results of an analysis. Chapter 3 defined the cost-effectiveness ratio, including the specific elements that went into its calculation in a

7. For example, in his foreword to *Healthy People*, a report published by the Department of Health and Human Services in 1979, President Jimmy Carter wrote that prevention "can substantially reduce both the suffering of our people and the burden on our expensive system of medical care." *Healthy People: The Surgeon General's Report on Health Promotion and Disease Prevention* (GPO, 1979).

study of drug treatment for hypertension. Chapter 4 discussed how to design an evaluation of exercise. Each of the chapters brought out the variations necessary to apply cost-effectiveness analysis to particular situations and some of the questions and controversies that are natural to a method that is still evolving.

The central purpose of cost-effectiveness analysis is to compare alternatives. Each study of a specific kind of prevention examines a set of alternatives. The study may compare a preventive program with the alternative of no program, as in the measles vaccine study. Or it may include a large number of alternatives—alternative assumptions about health effects, about costs, about the scope of the effort, and so on—as in the study of drug treatment for hypertension. These alternatives are evaluated using the same data and the same assumptions for factors that are not of direct interest for the comparison. Further, a study can evaluate alternative types of prevention as ways to improve health or it can compare methods for persuading people to adopt a particular method. Both are legitimate issues for evaluation, but the second logically follows the first; since the ultimate goal is better health, the cost-effectiveness of persuasion depends in large part on the cost-effectiveness of the measure as a way to improve health.

Most studies have focused on very specific issues. Is a program of measles vaccination a good investment? How about drugs to combat hypertension? Or tests to screen for cancer? These issues are important and some studies have had a major impact on the decisions made about them. Eddy's evaluation of screening tests for cancer is a notable example: the results of that analysis persuaded the American Cancer Society to recommend that tests be done less frequently than had been the case and that they be more carefully targeted to the age-groups at greatest risk. Cost-effectiveness analyses have also influenced the decision by Congress to pay for pneumococcal vaccine under medicare and some of the recommendations for using vaccines of the national Immunization Practices Advisory Committee.[8]

But cost-effectiveness analysis is also capable of helping with decisions across a wider range of choices—between different kinds of

8. For example, the committee published guidelines based on cost-effectiveness analysis to show when it saves money to screen for people who are already immune before administering hepatitis B virus vaccine. See "Recommendations of the Immunization Practices Advisory Committee (ACIP): Inactivated Hepatitis B Virus Vaccine," *Morbidity and Mortality Weekly Report*, vol. 31 (June 25, 1982), pp. 317–28.

prevention, between prevention and therapy, and between different methods of therapy—and the time is right to develop this capability. The rapid growth in medical expenditures during the 1960s and 1970s has been slowed in the 1980s, and medical care decisionmakers are increasingly subject to limits on the resources available to them. Hospital payments are limited under medicare, and some states have applied limits to all payers. All states, struggling with the growth in expenditures for medicaid, have placed limits on the payments made by their programs. Private employers are taking steps to slow the rise in their expenditures for medical care. Faced with these constraints, doctors, patients, and hospital administrators must try to choose those outlays that will bring the greatest improvement in health.

If cost-effectiveness analysis is to help make these decisions by allowing the wider range of comparisons they require, it must become more standardized. It would clearly be efficient if different studies subscribed to a common set of assumptions and a common approach wherever possible. At present, however, studies vary too much in approach and assumptions to permit comparisons between them.

A number of points could be standardized between studies without compromising analysts' freedom to represent the special characteristics of their problem. Six items in particular, already discussed in the preceding chapters, are suggested here for standardization: the perspective of the study; the discount rate; medical care costs in added years of life; the measurement of costs of institutionalization; the use of the year of healthy life as a measure of health effects; and the presentation of estimates of future earnings. Several other items, which for various reasons are not so easily standardized, are also discussed.

It is the practice in cost-effectiveness analysis to define a base case, a case that incorporates the most likely values for each variable. The proposals for each of the six issues essentially contribute to the definition of a standard base case. As they do now, individual studies could also present results for other cases that seemed useful, but the base case of any study would be comparable with the base case of any other study because all would share a common core of assumptions and methods.

Perspective of the Study

For comparability, different studies should adopt the same perspective. As noted in chapter 4, most studies in the literature take the social perspective, that is, they measure all the costs and effects of a preventive program, regardless of who pays them or who is affected. Only studies done from the social perspective show the overall costs and gains of a program. As a consequence, only studies done from the social perspective can support such general statements as "prevention does/does not save money," or "prevention is/is not a better investment than curative care." But by the same token, the results do not represent the costs and gains that will accrue to any subgroup of society—individuals, employers, or government programs.

Given that the social perspective does not represent any particular group's point of view, why should it be the dominant approach, the approach used for the standard base case? There are two reasons. First, no other perspective has a claim as *the* right perspective; any other perspective represents only one part of society. Second, there is great value from the point of view of policy in beginning with a perspective that includes *all* costs and effects, and that does not treat as a gain what is really only some other group's loss. The social perspective should be the touchstone. Studies may branch out from that societal starting point if the authors want to examine narrower perspectives.

Some studies will continue to be done from other perspectives. Government programs, employers, health insurers, and individuals want to know the benefits and costs that accrue specifically to them and will not always be willing to undertake the additional trouble and expense to analyze the benefits and costs for society. The authors of such studies should be clear in stating their point of view and the limitations of that point of view. They should scrupulously avoid statements suggesting that what is a good investment for a program, employer, insurer, or individual is necessarily a good investment for society because, again, the gains by the group in question may be offset by losses to other groups.

Discount Rate

All studies should use the same discount rate, or rates, for the base case. The discount rate can have a major effect on the results of a cost-effectiveness study and it is impossible to make valid comparisons between studies that use different discount rates. Cretin demonstrated that the effect of discounting can be particularly important for prevention, since it often does not produce benefits until many years after the costs have been incurred.[9]

9. Cretin, "Cost/Benefit Analysis of Treatment and Prevention of Myocardial Infarction," pp. 184–87.

Most studies in the literature use 4, 5, or 6 percent.[10] No one has suggested why one of these rates should be considered superior to the others, and they are too close to signal any real disagreement on the appropriate discount rate. It should therefore be relatively easy to reach agreement on 5 percent as the standard rate. If two standard rates are acceptable, zero should be the second one; as the extreme case of no discounting, zero shows how much the results can change as the discount rate is reduced and suggests whether the value judgment implicit in the discount rate is important for those results. If individual analysts prefer rates other than 5 or zero, they can, of course, report the results for those in addition to the standard rates.

Medical Costs in Added Years of Life

All studies estimate the medical costs associated with a preventive measure and any savings because disease is prevented. Some studies also include the medical expenses that would be incurred because a person lives longer. If the issue is how prevention will affect total expenditures for medical care, then medical expenditures in the years of life added by a preventive measure should be included in costs. But as was discussed in chapter 2, this is a narrow question, one that does not truly reflect society's perspective. When the question is instead simply whether the proposed program is a good use of society's resources, its indirect effects on medical expenditures are no more relevant than its indirect effects on expenditures for food, clothes, or housing.

Thus the estimates for the base case should exclude medical expenditures in added years of life. Because of the widespread interest in the effect of prevention on total expenditures for medical care, many analysts will want to make estimates including them as well, but these estimates should be identified as relevant only to the narrower question. Over the long run, the calculation including medical expenditures in added years of life should become less interesting as people are persuaded that prevention is rarely a free good.

Costs of Institutionalization

Again, the social perspective dictates that only the costs of institutionalization over and above the costs if the same person lived at home

---

10. These are real rates of discount, that is, rates after adjustment for inflation.

should be counted; the rest are matched by savings elsewhere in the economy. Similarly, the relevant costs of special education are the costs over and above those for a normal education. Most analysts are well aware of this, but the error does appear in some studies; it can lead to a substantial overestimate of the savings from preventing disease. Eliminating this error should be one of the easiest steps toward standardizing cost-effectiveness studies.

Measures of Health Effects

If studies are to be comparable, they must use the same measure of effects, and to accommodate all studies (as well as the way people actually judge health), that measure must allow for changes in the quality as well as the quantity of life. The year of healthy life, or quality-adjusted life-year, described in chapter 3 offers a practical way to accommodate these needs. The concept requires that individuals value states of health on a scale from zero to 1, where 1 is the value of a year of perfect health. When a preventive measure improves health or, because of side effects, makes it worse, the value of those gains and losses can then be calculated and summed to give the number of years of healthy life produced by the measure. The method permits the comparison of very different kinds of improvements in health and is a substantial advance over measures that make no allowance for changes in quality of life.

Although considerable progress has been made in its development, the year of healthy life is still a new idea and more work is needed if it is to serve as a true standard. In particular, consistent sets of weights need to be developed for use in different studies so that, for example, side effects from hypertension medication are not overweighted (or underweighted) relative to the quality of life with angina. Several researchers have shown that such weights can be developed. For example, the results of sample surveys conducted by Kaplan and Bush can serve as a direct source of weights for some studies and as a benchmark for the weights needed for studies of conditions that are not as well represented in those surveys.

Future Earnings

In some studies the authors calculate both the gains in health due to a preventive measure and the earnings made possible by those gains. If a cost-effectiveness ratio is calculated, they may subtract earnings from costs to yield net costs. More often, they simply suggest that earnings should be considered an offset to costs.

In general, however, it is incorrect to subtract earnings from costs because it amounts to double-counting some of the health effects. This is clear if one considers why gains in health are valuable. They are valuable partly *because* more and healthier people add to the output of the economy. To subtract gains in earnings from costs thus amounts to counting the same health benefit twice, once as a gain in years of life, and again as a saving to be subtracted from program costs. Further, this double-counting leads part of the way back to the position of cost-benefit analyses that use earnings to represent the value of health gains, a position many people rightly reject. Like those studies, subtracting earnings from costs in a cost-effectiveness study favors health gains for working people over gains for retired people or children.

Instead, earnings estimates should be viewed as providing additional detail about the health effects. They are one of the products for which the extra health can be used, along with time spent at school, time spent caring for children and other family members, and time spent in other productive and pleasant activities. Studies that include estimates of earnings should be careful to make it clear that earnings are not an addition to the health effects, only an amplification. If paid work is then favored over other activities in the decision about a preventive measure, the choice will be explicit and not hidden in the calculations.

Other Issues

Other issues can affect the comparability of different studies, some-times seriously. The four discussed below should prove more difficult to standardize than the first six—either because a good solution is not available or because the solution is difficult and expensive. They are offered here as an agenda for future discussion.

First, a good deal has been said in this study about the need to consider all the costs and effects of a measure, and it was noted at the beginning of the chapter that many authors limit themselves to estimating medical costs. The problem is that, desirable as it would be to go beyond medical care, it is difficult to do. For example, not much is known about how often certain conditions lead to dependency among the elderly, or how often a measure might prevent that dependency. Yet without such information, it is impossible to estimate whether there might be savings. The goal should be kept in mind, but in many cases it may be unattainable.

Second, chapter 4 discussed the fact that some preventive measures can make substantial use of the individual's time. Even when nobody pays for it, time represents a real resource and a limited one. Whenever the measure being studied requires a substantial amount of time, some attempt must be made to estimate the amount or the analysis will seriously understate the use of resources. The problem is that there is no accepted way to value the time in dollars so that it can be combined with other costs. Crude attempts to value it, while useful for individual studies, may distort comparisons between studies.

Third, studies of prevention often assume that not all patients comply with the prescribed regimen, while studies of curative care usually assume full compliance. But compliance is a problem for all forms of prevention and treatment; a study of a second-opinion program found that, even when two doctors agreed that surgery was indicated, almost a quarter of the patients declined it.[11] Perhaps the most practical solution would be to assume full compliance in the base case. The problem is that achieving full compliance in reality could involve substantial costs, the costs necessary to induce the most reluctant people to participate.[12] Thus imposing the assumption of full compliance will make some measures look hopelessly expensive. But it is not clear what lower level of compliance could serve as a standard.

Finally, it would be useful to have a sense of the degree of imprecision of the estimates presented in a study. A method for generating standard deviations was described in chapter 4. The problem is that it requires a large number of computer runs and is therefore expensive.

THE growing emphasis on cost containment in medical care makes it essential to have more and better information about the cost-effectiveness of different kinds of prevention, for different people, in different settings. As the growth in expenditures is slowed, decisions about allocating resources to particular investments will become more difficult.

11. Madelon L. Finkel, Hirsch S. Ruchlin, and Susan K. Parsons, *Eight Years' Experience with a Second Opinion Elective Surgery Program: Utilization and Economic Analyses*, Department of Health and Human Services, Health Care Financing Administration (Baltimore, Md.: HHS, 1981), p. 41.

12. Roy Shephard pointed out this problem during the discussion at the Ciba Symposium on the Value of Preventive Medicine on April 10–12, 1984, in London.

At the same time, it is more important than ever to channel resources to the programs and measures that can do the most for health. Cost-effectiveness analysis, done well and applied to both prevention and therapy, will help ensure that prevention receives a reasonable share of resources and that those resources are allocated to the most efficacious preventive programs.

Patricia J. Regan

appendix **Federally Funded Preventive Health Programs**

This appendix identifies and briefly describes federally funded preventive health programs as they stood in early 1985. The preventive programs outlined here are not a complete index of all federally funded preventive health services. Such an index would be very difficult to compile, since the preventive components of many programs are not reported individually. For example, only a small portion of the services paid for by medicare and medicaid are directed toward prevention or early screening, and these are not separately reported. This appendix does provide, however, a broad overview of the types of agencies and programs involved in disease prevention and health promotion. They are divided into two groups—programs within the Department of Health and Human Services (HHS) and programs run by other federal agencies. Budget obligations are shown in all tables presented in this appendix because outlay data for the separate programs are not available.

Preventive Programs within HHS

A number of smaller health programs, many of them directed at prevention, are the responsibility of the Public Health Service, a component of HHS. The organization of these programs was revised according to guidelines set out by the Omnibus Budget Reconciliation Act of 1981.[1] Under this act, twenty-two Public Health Service categorical grants were consolidated into four broad categories within HHS. That is, instead of states receiving separate federal grants for individual programs, each now receives a single federal grant for a group of programs.

1. Omnibus Budget Reconciliation Act of 1981, 95 Stat. 357, title 9.

Table A-1. Budget Obligations for HHS Health Block Grants, Fiscal Years 1982–85
Thousands of dollars

Block	1982 (actual)	1983 (actual)	1984 (actual)	1985 (estimated)
Alcohol, drug abuse, and mental health	428,095	468,000	462,000	490,000
Primary care	448,578	525,288	536,442	565,100
Maternal and child health	373,706	477,859	398,964	478,000
Preventive health and health services	81,600	86,300	88,187	89,500

Sources: *The Budget of the United States Government, Fiscal Year 1984—Appendix,* pp. I-K3, I-K10, I-K23, I-K26; *Fiscal Year 1985—Appendix,* pp. I-K3, I-K9, I-K21, I-K23; and *Fiscal Year 1986—Appendix,* pp. I-K3, I-K10, I-K22.

Each state then spends its block grant according to the purposes and conditions specified by the act.[2] Clearly, under this new legislation individual states have more flexibility in distributing funds to programs within each block and so can coordinate health services in ways most suited to their individual needs. This shifting of authority is an offshoot of the Reagan administration's "new federalism," designed to reestablish a more equal balance of power among federal, state, and local governments.[3]

The HHS block grants are designated by the following titles: alcohol, drug abuse, and mental health (ADAMH); primary care; maternal and child health; and preventive health and health services. Budget obligations for each block for 1982–85 are displayed in table A-1. A state match of 75 cents per federal dollar is required for the maternal and child health block, but no state match is required for any of the other blocks.

The preventive health and health services block is obviously the most purely preventive effort on the part of the federal government. The Public Health Service categorical grants consolidated to form this block were health incentive grants and those for high blood pressure, risk reduction and health education, fluoridation, rat control, home health services, emergency medical services, and rape crisis centers.[4] Since

2. *Review of 1981 Block Grants,* Hearings before the Senate Committee on Governmental Affairs, 97 Cong. 1 sess. (Government Printing Office, 1982), pp. 11–12.
3. *The Budget of the United States Government, Fiscal Year 1983,* p. 5-134; and Claude E. Barfield, *Rethinking Federalism: Block Grants and Federal, State, and Local Responsibilities* (Washington, D.C.: American Enterprise Institute for Public Policy Research, 1981), p. 35.
4. See Barfield, *Rethinking Federalism,* p. 84; and *Review of 1981 Block Grants,* p. 12.

1982 this block has been administered by the Centers for Disease Control (CDC). States are allowed to use up to 7 percent of this block grant for other HHS block grant programs.[5]

The other blocks also include some preventive programs, although they are not specifically identified as such. In the alcohol, drug abuse, and mental health block, at least 20 percent of the total funds must be used for prevention and early intervention.[6] The maternal and child health block, which includes a wide range of programs, works to reduce infant and maternal mortality through improved prenatal care services. Other goals—the prevention and reduction of unwanted pregnancies, of conditions leading to crippling, and of mental retardation—are administered through such programs as family planning services (including an adolescent family life program), a lead paint poisoning prevention program, and early screening and treatment for vision and hearing problems.[7] Both of these blocks, as well as the primary care block, become the responsibility of the Office of the Assistant Secretary for Health (HHS) in fiscal year 1985. In fiscal years 1982 through 1984, the ADAMH block was run by the Alcohol, Drug Abuse, and Mental Health Administration, while the maternal and child health and primary care blocks were run by the Health Resources and Services Administration.

Not all preventive health services provided through the Public Health Service are encompassed by the health block grants. The Centers for Disease Control administers several other preventive programs that were retained as categorical grants (see table A-2).

The goal of the venereal diseases program is to develop preventive and diagnostic techniques to reduce the number of cases and complications. State and local health agencies receive financial and technical assistance from the CDC. Financial assistance is in the form of grants, while technical assistance comprises training, laboratory backup, and operational research. (These methods of technical assistance are used for all CDC preventive programs.) State agencies use education, information, and service measures to lower the incidence of venereal diseases.

The infectious disease prevention program and the epidemic services program both work to reduce the occurrence of disease through improved preventive and diagnostic techniques. The CDC assists state and local

5. *Review of 1981 Block Grants*, p. 12.
6. Barfield, *Rethinking Federalism*, p. 31.
7. Karen Davis and Cathy Schoen, *Health and the War on Poverty: A Ten-Year Appraisal* (Brookings, 1978), p. 126.

Table A-2. Budget Obligations for Categorical Preventive Programs under the Centers for Disease Control, Fiscal Years 1982–85

Thousands of dollars

Program	1982 (actual)	1983 (actual)	1984 (actual)	1985 (estimated)
Sexually transmitted diseases	42,902	47,687	54,688	54,745
Infectious disease prevention	21,693	34,343	51,633	57,707
Epidemic services	29,930	37,354	47,554	48,931
Immunizations	34,715	39,253	42,068	54,277
Chronic and environmental disease prevention	27,055	31,389	25,953	28,568
Occupational Safety and Health (NIOSH)	62,058	57,469	65,872	66,173
Buildings and facilities	2,499	9,010	1,051	26,220
Program management	2,583	2,780	3,018	3,042

Sources: *The Budget of the United States Government, Fiscal Year 1984—Appendix*, p. I-K10; *Fiscal Year 1985—Appendix*, p. I-K9; and *Fiscal Year 1986—Appendix*, p. I-K10.

agencies in investigating the outbreak of any infectious or epidemic disease by lending personnel and providing technical assistance. Through national surveillance systems and quarantine programs, these two services prevent diseases from entering the United States from abroad.

Immunization services target the elimination of poliomyelitis, measles, rubella, mumps, diphtheria, pertussis (whooping cough), and tetanus. The CDC administers a grant program for state and local health agencies to carry on immunization programs aimed at both preschool and elementary school children. State and local agencies also receive CDC technical assistance and help in making sure that as many children as possible receive this series of immunizations.

The chronic and environmental disease prevention program focuses on controlling chronic diseases, reducing certain associated complications, and lessening the impact of environmental hazards on health. For example, this program helps curtail complications associated with diabetes through glucose and diet control measures. The CDC administers primarily technical assistance, but also some financial assistance, to state and local health agencies.

The National Institute of Occupational Safety and Health (NIOSH) of the CDC is involved in extensive research on causes of and cures for occupational diseases. The institute's findings are then used by the Occupational Safety and Health Administration (OSHA) and the Mine

Safety and Health Administration (MSHA), both in the Department of Labor, to set safety standards for places of work.[8]

There are other programs within HHS that work toward disease prevention and health promotion but are not grouped with the reported preventive health programs. The Food and Drug Administration, whose main job is to conduct research on the safety and efficacy of food, drugs, and consumer products, has undertaken a "sodium reduction initiative," encouraging lower sodium consumption in the hope of controlling hypertension.[9] The National Institutes of Health, consisting of ten biomedical research institutions and a number of management divisions and related research institutions, is establishing a new prevention unit under the Office of the Director. The new unit will act to "coordinate activities and set priorities in preventive research."[10]

Medicare and medicaid, both administered by the Health Care Financing Administration, are the two largest federal health programs, constituting almost 90 percent of total federal outlays for health. In fiscal year 1984 alone, federal outlays for medicare were $57.5 billion and for medicaid were $20.1 billion.[11] Medicaid is a joint federal and state program covering people on welfare. All states participating in medicaid are required to provide early and periodic screening, diagnosis, and treatment for recipients under age 21.[12] This preventive service covers screening and diagnosis to determine physical or mental defects, and treatment to correct any conditions discovered. Medicaid also pays for services that are usually considered preventive—such as visits to doctors and tests involved in treating hypertension. Medicare, a completely federal program benefiting the elderly and disabled, pays for these services as well but is prohibited by law from paying for routine preventive services such as physicals or immunizations (with the exception of pneumococcal pneumonia vaccine).[13]

8. Department of Health and Human Services, *Prevention '80*, DHHS (PHS) 81-50157 (HHS, 1980), p. 75.

9. *Budget Issues for Fiscal Year 1983*, Hearings before the House Committee on the Budget, 97 Cong. 2 sess. (GPO, 1982), vol. 1, p. 513.

10. Ibid., p. 518.

11. *The Budget of the United States Government, Fiscal Year 1986*, pp. 5-105, 5-111.

12. Department of Health and Human Services, Health Care Financing Administration, *The Medicare and Medicaid Data Book, 1981*, Health Care Financing Program Statistics, HCFA 03128 (HHS, 1982), p. 74.

13. Office of Technology Assessment, *A Review of Selected Federal Vaccine and Immunization Policies: Based on Case Studies of Pneumococcal Vaccine* (GPO,

Table A-3. Budget Obligations for USDA Food and Nutrition Service Programs, Fiscal Years 1982–85

Thousands of dollars

Program	1982 (actual)	1983 (actual)	1984 (actual)	1985 (estimated)
Food stamps	11,059,411	11,837,702	11,611,621	11,454,728
Child nutrition	2,884,101	3,295,193	3,556,606	3,809,418
Special supplemental food for WIC	929,436	1,218,184	1,366,617	1,423,757
Food donations	120,944	155,554	162,090	161,102
Special milk	19,520	19,435	18,632	17,321

Sources: *The Budget of the United States Government, Fiscal Year 1984—Appendix*, pp. I-E91 to I-E94; *Fiscal Year 1985—Appendix*, pp. I-E79 to I-E81; and *Fiscal Year 1986—Appendix*, pp. I-E88 to I-E92.

Programs Administered by Other Federal Agencies

HHS is only one among several federal departments making an effort to improve the population's health through prevention-oriented services. The U.S. Department of Agriculture (USDA) administers several nutrition programs aimed at promoting health by assuring the correct daily nutritional intake. The department's Food and Nutrition Service runs the food stamp program, the child nutrition program, the special supplemental food program for women, infants, and children, the food donations program, and the special milk program (see table A-3). Although these nutrition services are not necessarily preventive in each case, some of the recipients would not have a nutritionally sound diet without them.

The entire cost of the food stamp program is assumed by the federal government. State welfare agencies are responsible for certifying eligible households (based on household size and income) and for distributing the correct amount of stamps to each.

Federal assistance for the child nutrition program is administered through state agencies. Types of assistance provided are school lunches, school breakfasts, summer feeding, and child care feeding. The programs are authorized by the National School Lunch Act and the Child Nutrition Act of 1966.

The special supplemental food program for women, infants, and children is a federally subsidized program designed to provide nutritious

1979). The exception was enacted in 1980. 94 Stat. 3566 (amending title 18 of the Social Security Act).

Table A-4. Budget Obligations for the Occupational Safety and Health Administration
and the Mine Safety and Health Administration, Fiscal Years 1982–85

Thousands of dollars

Agency	1982 (actual)	1983 (actual)	1984 (actual)	1985 (estimated)
Occupational Safety and Health Administration				
Safety and health standards	6,442	6,070	5,910	6,250
Enforcement				
Federal enforcement	74,693	80,111	84,807	84,118
State programs	47,238	50,248	49,620	53,021
Compliance assistance	37,940	37,013	35,857	37,856
Mine Safety and Health Administration				
Enforcement				
Coal	64,707	75,031	76,220	76,364
Metal-nonmetal	27,191	27,367	29,056	29,936
Standards development	688	725	886	895
Assessments	3,934	2,154	2,031	1,908
Educational policy and development	12,246	11,899	11,923	11,910

Sources: *The Budget of the United States Government, Fiscal Year 1984—Appendix*, pp. I-017, I-018; *Fiscal Year 1985—Appendix*, pp. I-018, I-019; and *Fiscal Year 1986—Appendix*, pp. I-017, I-018.

foods to pregnant women, recent mothers, infants, and children who do not otherwise receive the recommended daily nutritional intake.

The food donations program provides commodities instead of stamps to eligible families (mainly on Indian reservations and in the Pacific Trust Territory). The commodities are purchased by the Commodity Credit Corporation, which is later reimbursed with federal funds. This program also provides subsidies for programs to feed the elderly.

The special milk program encourages the consumption of milk in schools and institutions that do not normally participate in other federally subsidized meal programs. State agencies distribute the milk and then file claims for federal reimbursement.

The Department of Labor also implements preventive services. The Occupational Safety and Health Administration and the Mine Safety and Health Administration, both within the Labor Department's jurisdiction, concentrate on setting safety and health standards based on NIOSH research as discussed earlier, and on their own experience and review of existing standards (see table A-4). Enforcement of these standards takes two principal forms—physical inspections and compliance assistance. OSHA conducts inspections of facilities and encourages employers to initiate voluntary labor-management self-inspection programs. Compliance assistance promotes cooperative agreements, through

Table A-5. Environmental Protection Agency Budget Obligations for Abatement, Control, and Compliance Programs, Fiscal Years 1982–85

Thousands of dollars

Program	1982 (actual)	1983 (actual)	1984 (actual)	1985 (estimated)
Air quality	116,290	108,104	113,280	110,027
Water quality	116,798	107,112	114,086	135,187
Drinking water	40,944	39,621	40,189	43,217
Hazardous waste	61,426	63,185	67,884	103,843
Pesticides	24,411	22,253	21,344	29,225
Toxic substances	27,988	22,506	23,355	67,112
Radiation	2,987	3,843	2,974	2,284

Sources: *The Budget of the United States Government, Fiscal Year 1984–Appendix*, p. I-S3; *Fiscal Year 1985—Appendix*, p. I-S3; and *Fiscal Year 1986—Appendix*, p. I-S3.

which states are reimbursed for 90 percent of the costs involved in providing free on-site consultations to employers at their request. Also included in compliance assistance are grants to organizations to help them develop their abilities to provide occupational safety and health training for employers and employees. MSHA also enforces its standards through inspections and on-site education and training assistance. Investigations are always made of serious mine accidents, with the aim of preventing similar occurrences. Assessments of civil monetary penalties are made in the case of violations of the set standards.

The Environmental Protection Agency (EPA) is another federal agency that devotes many of its energies to services that are preventive. The agency protects the population's health by regulating actions that could be detrimental to the environment. Abatement and control programs that help prevent any deterioration in the environment's quality are shown in table A-5. These activities are carried out through contracts, grants, and cooperative agreements.

Each of these EPA programs involves federal and state cooperation in the setting of quality standards and the writing of regulations and guidelines. The first three programs listed in the table are directed toward maintaining air and water quality and controlling hazardous waste. The pesticides program requires the review and registration of all pesticide products, and the toxic substances program requires the evaluation and control of all new and existing chemicals. Finally, the radiation program works to reduce exposure to both ionizing and nonionizing radiation sources.

The EPA provides financial and technical assistance to state and local agencies to help them meet the standards and execute the regulations and guidelines. When the state or local agency is unable to meet the requirements of the air quality program, the federal government will itself take direct action. Nonregulatory approaches to compliance with the toxic substances program are used when necessary.

Finally, the National Highway Traffic Safety Administration (NHTSA), a part of the Department of Transportation, administers several highway traffic safety programs. The administration provides technical assistance to states for the planning and implementation of these programs. Types of programs supported are demonstration programs for alcohol countermeasures and safety belt usage, the Presidential Commission on Drunk Driving, and child passenger information services. The goal of each is to reduce highway injuries and fatalities. Budget obligations for NHTSA highway traffic safety grants were $97 million in fiscal years 1982 and 1983, $106 million in fiscal year 1984, and an estimated $155 million for 1985.[14]

14. *The Budget of the United States Government, Fiscal Year 1984—Appendix,* p. I-Q12; *Fiscal Year 1985—Appendix,* p. I-Q12; and *Fiscal Year 1986—Appendix,* p. I-Q14.

Index

Abel-Smith, Brian, 2n
Acres, S. E., 25n, 28n
Added years of life. *See* Year of healthy life
Adjaye, Nellie, 40n
Age-varying partial benefit assumption, 73, 74
Albritton, Robert B., 24n
Alderslade, R., 3n, 39n
Amery, Antoon, 43n, 47n, 56n
Anderson, Roy M., 26n
Arita, I., 11n, 14n, 20n
Asbury, W., 12n
Atkins, Catherine J., 70n
Axnick, Norman W., 19n, 24n, 25n, 31n, 110n

Bahn, Anita K., 62n
Balance-sheet method, 31–37, 102–04
Barfield, Claude E., 122n, 123n
Belloc, Nedra B., 80n
Berg, Robert L., 33n, 67n
Bergner, Marilyn, 70n, 99n
Berkman, Lisa F., 81n
Berry, Charles C., 69n
Berwick, Donald M., 79n, 110n
Blair, Steven N., 86n, 90n, 91n
Brandling-Bennett, A. David, 26n
Brauer, Alan P., 61n
Brennan, P. J., 52n
Breslow, Lester, 80n, 81n
Brilliant, L. B., 21n, 22n
Brook, Robert H., 55n
Build and Blood Pressure studies, 46–47
Bush, J. W., 33n, 69, 117

Cancer screening, 61–62, 77–78, 98, 113
Cantu, Robert C., 91n
Carter, Jimmy, 2n, 112n
Chen, M. M., 33n
Cherry, James D., 25n, 26–27n
Christie, A. B., 10n, 14n, 23n
Cleary, Patricia, 87n
Cochrane, A. L., 61n

Cockburn, W. Charles, 19n
Colon cancer screening, 78
Compliance, 74–76, 119
Cost-benefit analysis, 14n, 30–31, 36
Cost-effectiveness analysis: balance-sheet method, 31–37, 102–04; cost-effectiveness ratio method, 71–76, 104, 118; defined, 5–6, 31; of exercise, 82, 91, 94–105; of hypertension screening and treatment, 4, 71–76, 97–98; of measles vaccination, 30–37, 97; perspective determination, 33, 72, 95–96, 104, 114–15; purpose, 113–14; standardization recommendations, 114–20
Costs: exercise, 90–94, 100–02; hypertension screening and treatment, 64–66, 71–76; institutionalization, 32–34, 116–17; measles vaccination, 30, 32–34, 37; smallpox vaccination, 18–19. *See also* Discounting; Medical costs in added years of life
Cretin, Shan, 79n, 106n, 110n, 111, 115
Cutting, W. A. M., 30n

Dauer, Carl C., 1n, 11n, 12n, 13n, 23n, 24n
Davies, J. W., 25n, 28n
Davis, Karen, 123n
Dawber, Thomas Royle, 43n, 44n, 45
Diagnostic testing, accuracy of, 51, 61–64
Discounting, 33–34, 73, 103, 115–16
Draper, W. F., 12–13n
Drummond, Michael F., 100n
Duffy, John, 11n, 12n

Eddy, David M., 41n, 62n, 66n, 76–79, 98, 113
Edwards, P., 86n
Enstrom, James E., 81n
Evans, J. G., 51n
Exercise: cost-effectiveness, 82, 91, 94–105; costs, 90–94, 100–02; health effects, 82–87, 97–100; recommended-level guides, 89–90

131

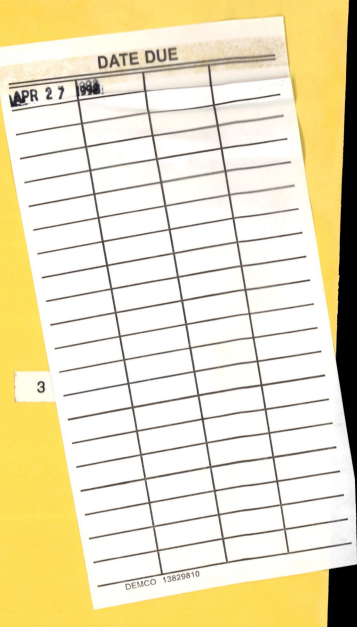

DATE DUE

APR 27 1998			

3